WARD LOCK

FAMILY HEALTH GUIDE

OSTEOPOROSIS

CLARE DOVER

IN ASSOCIATION WITH THE
NATIONAL OSTEOPOROSIS SOCIETY

WARD LOCK

Clare Dover
Clare Dover is an experienced journalist specializing in science and medicine. She has been Science Correspondent for the Daily Telegraph newspaper, and Medical Reporter for the Daily Express until 1993. She now works as a freelance medical journalist and lives in London.

A WARD LOCK BOOK

First published in the UK 1994
by Ward Lock
Villiers House
41/47 Strand
London
WC2N 5JE

A Cassell Imprint

Designed and produced
by SP Creative Design
147 Kings Road, Bury St Edmunds, Suffolk, England

Editor: Heather Thomas
Art Director: Rolando Ugolini
Illustrations: Rolando Ugolini

Distributed in the United States
by Sterling Publishing Co., Inc.
387 Park Avenue South, New York, NY 10016-8810

Distributed in Australia
by Capricorn Link(Australia) Pty Ltd
2/13 Carrington Road, Castle Hill, NSW 2154

A British Library Cataloguing in Publication Data block for this book may be obtained from the British Library.

ISBN 0 7063 7256 5

Printed and bound in Spain

Acknowledgements
The publishers and author would like to acknowledge the invaluable help given to them by the National Osteoporosis Society in producing this book.
Cover photograph: Comstock Photo Library
Adam Hart-Davis/Science Photo Library: page 29
Sandoz Pharmaceuticals: page 19
Mark Shearman: pages 28, 62
Sheila Terry/Science Photo Library: page 41

Contents

Introduction

The National Osteoporosis Society has raised awareness that osteoporosis is a major public health problem. It is important that each and everyone of us takes action now to protect our bones against this painful disease.

The NOS is very grateful to Clare Dover for her help in highlighting the seriousness of this cruel and very underestimated disease.

Please read this book, share it with your family and friends and take its recommendations to heart. It is only in this way that we can stem the rising tide of fractures.

Linda Evans
Director of the National Osteoporosis Society

More of us are living to a ripe old age, only to have our later years blighted by osteoporosis. For countless thousands of women, and men too, it is the unseen robber, which slowly erodes their skeletons while they are unaware of its ravages, and cheats them of their future good health.

Osteoporosis weakens the bones, distorts the skeleton and causes untold pain and discomfort. Sprightly people become bowed. A fall and a subsequent fractured wrist or hip may have disastrous consequences and affect the future quality of their lives.

A silent epidemic, osteoporosis is a growing scourge of our modern society. However, it is largely preventable, provided that we each take action to keep it at bay. This book will help show you how to do this. It is dedicated to everyone, men as well as women, whatever their age. It explains how to insure ourselves for a healthier future.

As a result of writing the book, I have modified my own lifestyle. I hope that you will, too.

Clare Dover

Chapter one

The silent epidemic

Osteoporosis is sometimes called the silent epidemic.Most women, and some men, who are affected by it are unaware of its onset and only realise their bones have become lightweight and fragile when they fall and break a wrist, or, worse still, fracture their hip. Their spine may become more curved and painful, and they are no longer as tall as they used to be. It becomes less easy to sit in a comfortable position, and clothes which used to fit perfectly start to pucker because of the so-called 'widow's hump'.

For years, it has been considered an inevitable part of ageing – a totally outdated notion in the light of modern medical knowledge. It is, in fact, largely preventable, and there are treatments that can help stop deterioration and alleviate the problems incurred. Prevention is realistic and could reduce much pain and expense and save many lives.

Good bones that should last a lifetime are begun in childhood. Peak bone mass is achieved by about the age of 30 or possibly 35. Bone loss related to age begins after that, slow at first, quicker later. In women, acceleration of bone loss caused by the menopause additionally exposes them to osteoporosis.

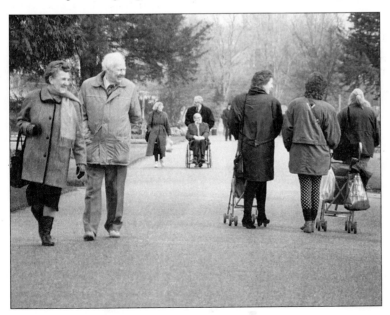

Most women do not notice the onset of osteoporosis until many years after menopause when bone loss is accelerated. Nowadays, it is possible to take preventive measures. Eating a good diet which is high in calcium and exercising regularly to keep your skeleton strong and healthy are both helpful.

The silent epidemic

Fractures

Osteoporosis literally means 'porous bones'. The bones have lost much of the calcium they need to remain strong and firm, and in this brittle state, a fall from which people would pick themselves up and nurse their bruises, results in fractures from which an elderly person may never properly recover. By the time fractures are occurring, the skeleton may have lost 30 per cent of the calcium that should be its source of strength. It can cause great disability, often accelerating death. There are three main types of fractures resulting from osteoporosis: hip, vertebral and Colles (wrist).

Sadly, many people are dying early because of osteoporosis, and many more are living their lives in disability, discomfort and pain. Instead of enjoying a healthy and active old age, their quality of life and ability to get around are drastically reduced. About a quarter of those who suffer a hip fracture die from it and about half lose their independence and became dependent on their families.

Osteoporosis fact

Osteoporosis affects one in four women over the age of 70. Men also suffer, but not to the same extent. One in 20 men are estimated to have brittle and porous bones. In the UK, there are currently two million women with osteoporosis, many of whom have seen their quality of life deteriorate through deformity and pain.

A working part of the Royal College of Physicians in the UK found that patients with hip fractures occupied 20 per cent of orthopedic beds in hospitals. Of these, 80 per cent were women aged over 65 years. Osteoporosis causes incalculable human misery and is a financial burden to the National Health Service in the UK. The annual hospital cost of treating the fractures and caring for the victims of fractured hips who often have to spend long periods in hospital is estimated at at least £640 million. And that is a conservative estimate, and rising year by year.

Between the ages of 70 and 80, one in four women and one in 40 men will have sustained a fracture related to osteoporosis. Although anyone at any age can take a tumble, the traumatic fractures would largely not have happened without the underlying causes. This is an important point, because in the past, the professional conception of osteoporosis has been hampered by the acceptance of the accidental cause rather than the bone weakness as the cause of fractures.

Strategies to prevent falls are important, but less so than strategies to prevent bone weakness in the first place.

Vertebral or spinal fractures can cause considerable pain. These are crush fractures of the vertebrae which have healed badly, with irreversible displacement. The resulting distortion of the spinal anatomy is often painful because of obstruction of the nerve

Common bone fractures

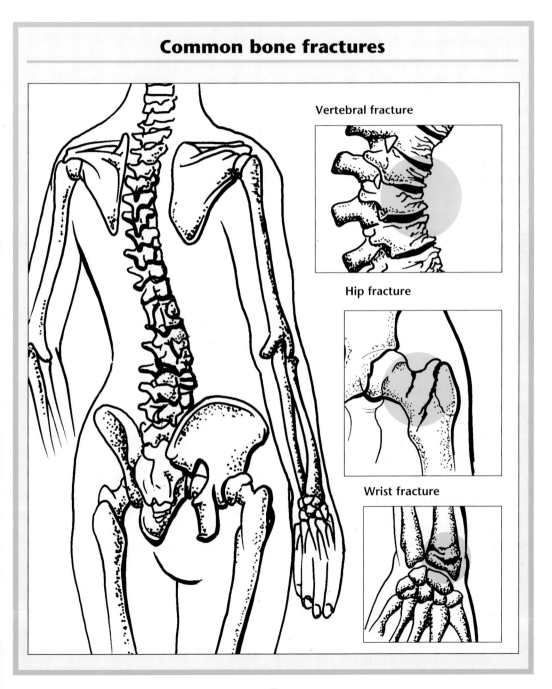

Vertebral fracture

Hip fracture

Wrist fracture

The silent epidemic

net. When several vertebrae have collapsed, there is a loss of height because of the shortening and compression of the spine. This reduces the capacity of the chest and abdominal cavities and interferes with the action of the heart, lungs, stomach and bladder and can cause difficulties in breathing, hiatus hernia and incontinence. The catalogue of suffering extends far beyond broken bones.

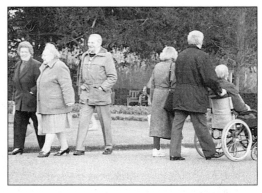

You can continue to lead a healthy life as you get older. Regular exercise, such as walking or playing golf, will help keep you fit and strong during and after the menopause. Build it into your everyday routine so that it becomes an enjoyable part of your life.

The increase in osteoporosis

Although it is thought of as a disease of old age, there are occasional sufferers in their twenties and thousands of women in their fifties are already affected.

The growth of the problem is truly alarming, with five times as many broken bones due to osteoporosis each year as there were in the 1960s. The Royal College of Physicians in the UK reports that the incidence of hip fractures rose 254 per cent between 1954 and 1983 and was then still rising, although there have since been some signs that it may be levelling off. Every ten minutes someone in the UK has a fracture.

Increasing numbers of elderly people in the population explain some of this increase, but they do not provide the whole explanation. Other aspects of our lifestyles have been contributing to the upsurge for which there is still no full explanation.

Possible causes of the upsurge

The modern pattern of a sedentary lifestyle with its emphasis on desk jobs rather than physical work, using the car rather than walking, and the lure of the television set which has replaced more active pursuits, could be factors in the shortfall in the amount of exercise we need to keep our skeletons strong and healthy.

Changes in diet have certainly made us taller than our ancestors, and research indicates that tall heavier people may be more prone to fractures when they fall than shorter people, but firm proof is lacking. It may have more to do with the mechanics of falling, and if the relationship is established, it is one more factor lacking an explanation.

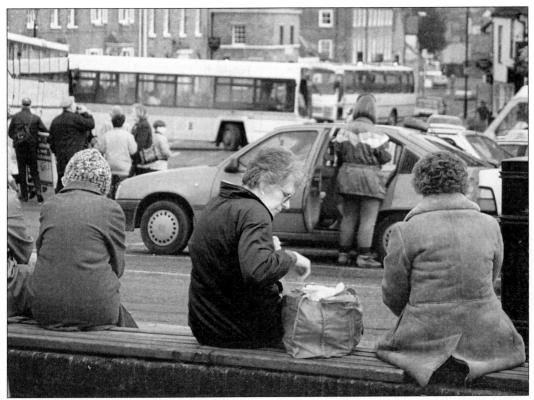

Researchers confess that they have only a vague understanding of how overall bone quality has deteriorated in current times, compared to the nineteenth century when many people were living in poverty, had never heard the phrase 'healthy lifestyle', and had diets that were often well

Today's modern sedentary lifestyle has probably contributed to the upsurge in osteoporosis. It is now more important than ever to eat a healthy diet and to exercise regularly.

below what would currently be considered optimum requirements.

Prevention and treatment

Although we may not know precisely what we are doing wrong, we do have some valuable pointers to help turn the tide. Whether they are young or old, male or female, everyone should be aware of osteoporosis because its prevention depends on adopting more healthy eating patterns and lifestyle throughout our lives, coupled with the

11

The silent epidemic

awareness to seek medical intervention before it has had a chance to progress.

The good news is that osteoporosis can be effectively treated and prevented in most people. To achieve this, we all need to protect our bones from childhood to old age.

The ambitious goal is to make osteoporosis a disease of the past. If this is to be achieved, it will mean that it must be given a higher priority by the medical profession. Many doctors learned little about it when they were studying medicine at medical school and are, like the general public, still in the process of learning about the importance

Menopause

The central problem for women comes at the menopause, when the hormone pattern changes. Loss of oestrogen, which used to be produced by the ovaries, has a knock-on effect on the quality of bone in every part of the skeleton, leading to bone loss which is inevitable and irrevocable unless action is taken against it.

of prevention and treatment. The National Osteoporosis Society in the UK has produced an information pack for doctors, to raise the level of medical education.

On their own, though, doctors cannot turn the tide for us. The current philosophy of individuals taking more responsibility for their own health, highlights the need for every person to know more about the condition and tackle prevention on an everyday basis in the way we live our lives. This includes knowing when to go to the doctor, rather than leaving a consultation until the condition has become advanced.

Exercise

Load-bearing exercise, such as going for brisk walks, is another important factor. It is never too late to start adopting good eating and exercise patterns, which, with hindsight, we should have embraced much earlier in our lives. Our bodies now need careful nurturing to preserve our bones against fractures.

Evolution and osteoporosis

Back in the dim and distant history of the evolution of the human race, mankind started out with much stronger and heavier skeletons which were better able to withstand the knocks and falls. When human life first emerged in the Rift Valley of

Africa 200,000 years ago, we came with skeletons which were heavy and dense and extremely powerful. However, as our ancestors migrated, moving up the globe into higher latitudes, genetic changes took place which caused a deterioration in the quality of the human skeleton. The European and other lighter skinned races became lighter boned. Why this happened is a total mystery.

It is a matter of interest to researchers that black women of African descent do not get osteoporosis with anything like the severity of white women. They are the inheritors of the original human skeleton.

During early childhood, the bone development of blacks and whites is almost identical, but in late puberty, while black children are laying down an additional 34 per cent of bone, white children are undergoing an average 11 per cent increase.

For Caucasian, Asian and Oriental women, the predisposition to osteoporosis is programmed in the genes, with women in some families running a higher risk than those in others. Having a close relative who has had osteoporosis should act as a warning if you are entering the age range when you could develop the condition. However, coming from a family in which bone problems have not featured prominently, is no guarantee of immunity.

Genes and osteoporosis

A gene that appears to play a crucial role in the development of osteoporosis has been discovered by researchers in Australia. It is the first major insight into the genetics of osteoporosis. A team led by Professor John Eisman at the Garvan Institute of Medical Research in Sydney has found that bone density is strongly influenced by a single gene. The single gene accounts for up to 75 per cent of the total genetic effect on bone density, excluding the influences of diet and lifestyle.

The gene carries a receptor for vitamin D, which affects the way the human body incorporates calcium into bone. These findings will have to confirmed by further research on a wider range of people. However, they open the way for the development of a genetic test to discover who is most at risk of developing osteoporosis.

Those people who are shown to be at risk could then be offered vitamin D treatment much earlier in life. Although the development of preventive treatment for osteoporosis resulting from this exciting discovery is still many years away, there is now hope of opening the route to developing improved methods of prevention and helping many people in the future.

Chapter two
Your skeleton

The skeleton is not a dead framework which holds the other parts of the body in place.

It is a living, changing structure which is constantly rebuilding and replacing itself, not just during our growing years but for the whole of the lifespan. Throughout our lives, old cells are being absorbed and got rid of, to be replaced by new cells, incorporating the calcium from our diet as its structural material, with exercise helping to ensure that the rebuilding programme is maintained.

The skeleton is also the storage system for calcium, so that if the body is not receiving enough for its other needs, it withdraws calcium from the skeleton to meet its other demands. This is why calcium is particularly important during pregnancy, as the growing unborn child will call on its mother's skeletal reserves if the calcium intake is insufficient to meet the demand.

Changes in bone mass

Most of our bone mass is accumulated during the first 20 years of life. There is then a phase of consolidation until the age of about 35. After that there is a period of bone loss in men and women. Typically there is a mismatch as creation of new bone lags behind the rate of bone loss. The result is one-half a per cent reduction in bone mass per year.

Rapid gain in bone mass occurs in infancy and adolescence in both sexes. In early childhood, males and females have similar bone mass but after puberty, males have a greater amount of the dense outer layer of bone than females. Between 85 and 90 per cent of the peak bone mass – the heaviest the bones ever become – is accumulated before the age of 20, with the remainder being achieved between the ages of 20 and 35 to 40 years. This is during the consolidation phase.

Between 1968 and 1971, birth records were individually linked to school health examination records, and this has helped medical researchers in looking back at the development of a group of women to see if any relationships can be established between the present quality of their bones and their development as children.

This prompted British researchers to trace and persuade 155 women born in the town of Bath between 1968 and 1969 to volunteer for bone examinations to and allow their childhood records to be opened. No relationship was found between their weight at birth and their bone mineral content and bone mass density at the age of 21. This suggests that any adverse influences

The human skeleton

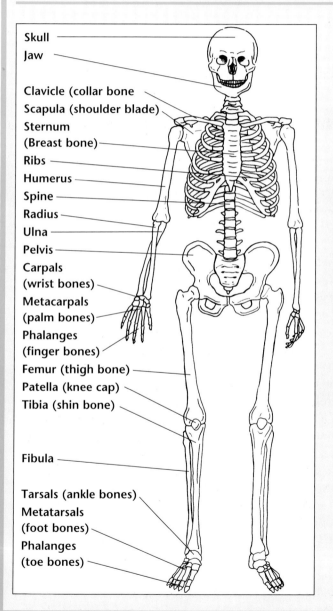

Skull

Jaw

Clavicle (collar bone

Scapula (shoulder blade)

Sternum
(Breast bone)

Ribs

Humerus

Spine

Radius

Ulna

Pelvis

Carpals
(wrist bones)

Metacarpals
(palm bones)

Phalanges
(finger bones)

Femur (thigh bone)

Patella (knee cap)

Tibia (shin bone)

Fibula

Tarsals (ankle bones)

Metatarsals
(foot bones)

Phalanges
(toe bones)

Your skeleton gives your body its shape and supports and protects it. There are 206 bones in the skeleton, which are made of living matter and are constantly being replaced with new material by their cells. If these cells remove more bone than they replace the bones become weak, and after the age of 35 our bones naturally start to lose some of the calcium that gives them their strength and density. The rate of bone loss accelerates around and following the menopause in women. The drop in the level of the female hormone oestrogen causes most osteoporosis.

15

Your skeleton

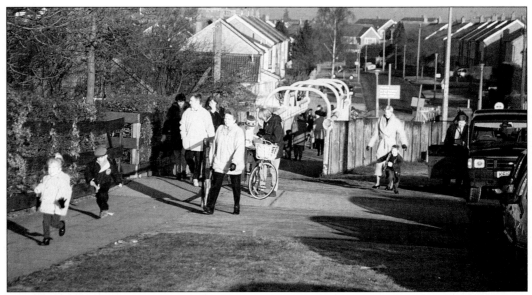

It is very important that children get adequate exercise. Walking to school instead of going by car, playing games, cycling and swimming all help to build stronger and healthier bones for later on in their adult lives.

at birth can be overcome. But the babies who had developed into the heaviest one-year-olds had the best quality bones with high mineral content at 21 years. This is a strong indicator of the importance of adequate nutrition during the first year of life. Their height at the age of ten and at 21 bore no relation to their bone mineral content as adults, and weight at the age of ten was only poorly related to bone outcome as adults.

However, measurements of the bone at the neck of the femur – the thigh bone which is the strongest bone in the body – did show a relationship with outdoor walking. Those who recalled doing a great deal of

walking when they were youngsters had developed the strongest thigh bones. There may be lessons here for the future that walking to school with your children may be giving them a better start in life than driving them there in the family car.

Building healthy bones

If researchers can identify the various factors involved in the building of healthy bone and the biological processes involved in bone depletion, there is hope of being able to influence the whole population. Unfortunately, specialists at the forefront of research admit that they are nowhere near to achieving any great understanding of the factors governing these processes.

Hormone control of calcium

It is thought that there is little need for people in Britain eating an average diet to take calcium supplements, although there may be a case for supplementing the amount of calcium in the very elderly.

The action of three hormones controls the calcium levels in the blood: parathyroid hormone, 1,25 dihydroxy-vitamin D and calcitonin. These hormones control the absorption of calcium by the intestine, its excretion by the kidneys and the uptake of calcium by the bone. About 30 per cent of the calcium in our diets is absorbed under normal circumstances, but the efficiency of its absorption varies, increasing during growth and pregnancy and at times of reduced intake.

Bone is constantly being broken down and rebuilt under hormone control, a process known as 'remodelling', which involves specialized bone cells. Cells called osteoblasts help in the laying down of new bone and others called osteoclasts are responsible for the resorption or removal of bone. The parathyroid hormone stimulates bone loss through resorption, and calcitonin inhibits this process. The sex hormones, growth

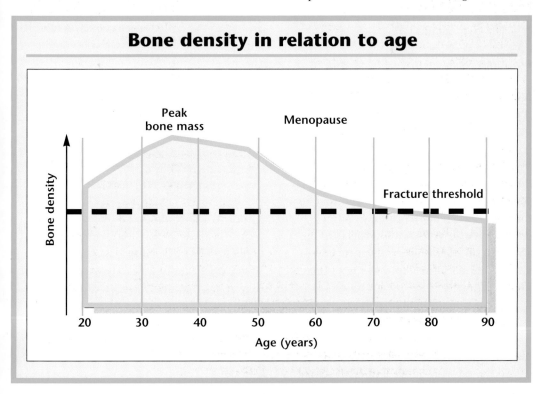

Bone density in relation to age

Peak bone mass

Menopause

Fracture threshold

Bone density

Age (years)

Your skeleton

hormone and other hormones also influence bone metabolism.

Bone has its own supply of blood vessels and, when•healthy, can withstand great stress and strain without fracturing. For example, youngsters can pick themselves up from falls that would have put an elderly person in hospital with complicated fractures.

When the rate of rebuilding fails to match the rate at which bone is breaking down, the skeleton becomes progressively depleted and weaker. This is the start of osteoporosis.

The onset of osteoporosis

From the outside, osteoporotic bones do not change visibly, but inside, the structure of the honeycomb mesh of cells from which bones derive their strength is slowly being broken down. The bones of the skeleton consist of:the following:

- A strong and densely packed outer casing called cortical bone.

- A mesh-like structure inside called trabecular bone.

In osteoporosis, the outer (cortical) bone is thinner and the inner (trabecular) bone is lighter and less densely packed. Under the microscope, the inner zone of osteoporotic bone appears flimsy and full of holes. Small areas within the bone become denuded of their former structural cells. Filled with holes and gaps, the bone loses its ability to absorb shock safely, and the flimsier it becomes, the greater is the risk of fracture when someone takes a fall.

The importance of exercise

Pulling of the muscles on the skeleton through exercise and activity keeps the skeleton strong and the bone responsive to the message to rebuild properly. Tennis players have heavier bones in their serving arm than on their non-serving side. Long-distance runners have sturdier spines than people who rarely take any exercise.

People who have built strong skeletons during their youth start from a better base when bone loss does occur. They literally have more to lose before entering the danger zone.

People who are active and take regular

Creating healthy children

- Encourage your child to play games rather than watch TV.
- Go for family walks.
- Go swimming with your child.
- Walk your child to school if possible.
- Give your child milk, yogurt, cheese and sardines to boost calcium intake.

Bone density

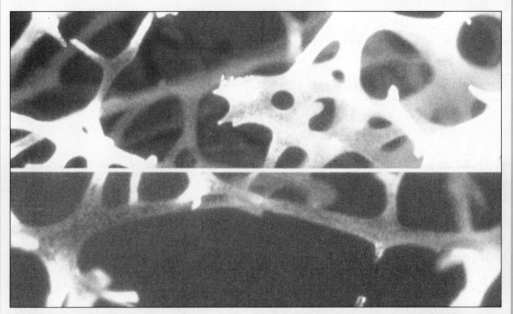

These micrograph pictures show the appearance of normal bone(top) and osteoporotic bone(below). The interior of normal bone is filled with cells, but in osteoporosis their density decreases. Thus the bones become less strong and more brittle, and are liable to fracture easily.

exercise have better quality bones overall than those who spend most of their lives sitting down. There is a message here for people in sedentary jobs to take a purposeful approach to exercise, whether through running, jogging, playing golf or some other form of sport. Try to build exercise into your everyday routine: walking where possible rather than taking the car, and use the stairs rather than the lift or escalator.

This health lesson is in line with the one being urged by 'healthy heart' educators, and gives us one more reason to take the exercise message seriously.

Watching television and playing video games are time-consuming pastimes for many of today's schoolchildren, and parents are often happy that they are safe indoors rather than at risk on the streets. However, *continued on page 21*

Your skeleton

Remodeling of bone surface

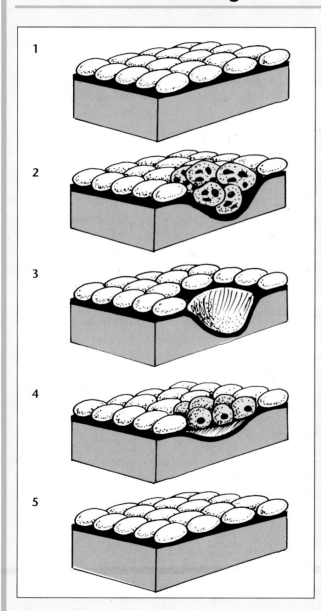

1 In the resting phase the surface of the bone is covered by a protective layer of bone cells.

2 During resorption, large cells with many nuclei, known as osteoclasts, invade and erode the bone surface, dissolving the mineral.

3 When resorption is complete, a small cavity made by osteoclasts is created in the surface of the bone.

4 The cavity is filled in with new bone, including collagen and minerals, by the bone-forming cells.

5 When the repair is completed, the surface of the bone is restored.

sports educators are concerned that the modern youngster is doing very little physically to raise a sweat in more energetic pursuits. They would like to see a better balance between the active and the sedentary use of free time. They also note that children who are keen on playing sport tend to continue this in their later life. The habits of a lifetime are often developed in childhood and are more difficult to change later, so encourage your children or grandchildren to be as active as possible. The important thing is to build up as much bone as possible when young through diet and exercise, so that when bone loss does start to occur, it is being lost from a substantial base.

Bone deterioration and primary osteoporosis

If unchecked, osteoporosis can make you become bowed and less tall than you used to be. Some people lose an inch or two in height. More severe cases can lose up to eight or nine inches. Loss of height occurs when the spinal column becomes more curved and the vertebrae crush together.

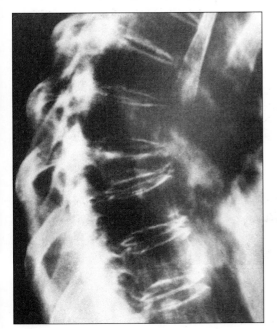

Spinal osteoporosis seems to affect mostly women aged between 50 and 60. The neck becomes weak and the head hangs forward. The bones of the spine crush together, and pain develops in part or all of the back. The development of back pain after the age of 50 can be a warning sign.

Primary osteoporosis, which most commonly occurs after the menopause, is so called because it is totally unrelated to any underlying condition, such as diabetes or rheumatoid arthritis, and has not been triggered as a side effect of corticosteroid drugs. In most cases, osteoporosis will have no apparent underlying cause.

Deformities of the spine include kyphosis (an outward curvature of the upper spine) and lordosis (an inward curvature of the lower spine).

Undetected progressive bone loss often manifests itself by one or more vertebral

This X-ray shows the spine of a woman who is suffering from osteoporosis. It shows the vertebral collapse from a reduction in bone mass resulting in a vertebral crush fracture.

Your skeleton

Vertebral fractures of the spine

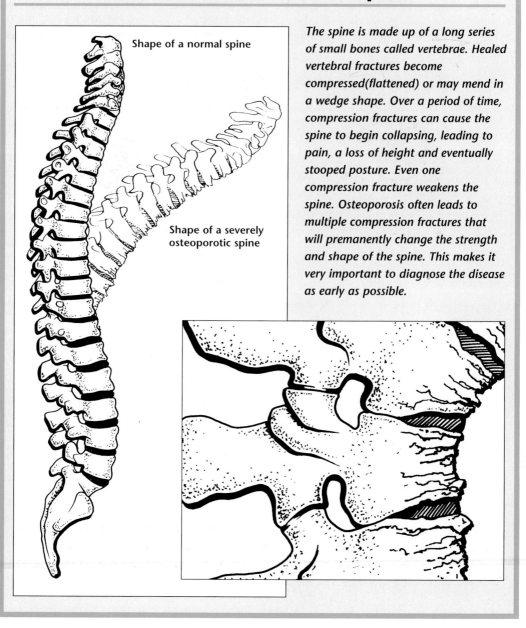

Shape of a normal spine

Shape of a severely osteoporotic spine

The spine is made up of a long series of small bones called vertebrae. Healed vertebral fractures become compressed(flattened) or may mend in a wedge shape. Over a period of time, compression fractures can cause the spine to begin collapsing, leading to pain, a loss of height and eventually stooped posture. Even one compression fracture weakens the spine. Osteoporosis often leads to multiple compression fractures that will premanently change the strength and shape of the spine. This makes it very important to diagnose the disease as early as possible.

fractures that result from the simple stresses of daily life being placed on fragile and weakened bones. Vertebral fractures can be caused by something as simple as lifting a bag of groceries, bending over to pick up a newspaper, or even just by sneezing.

Bone mass in adult women is usually less than that in men at a comparable age. In addition, women will experience a period of accelerated bone loss following the menopause.

Stooped posture

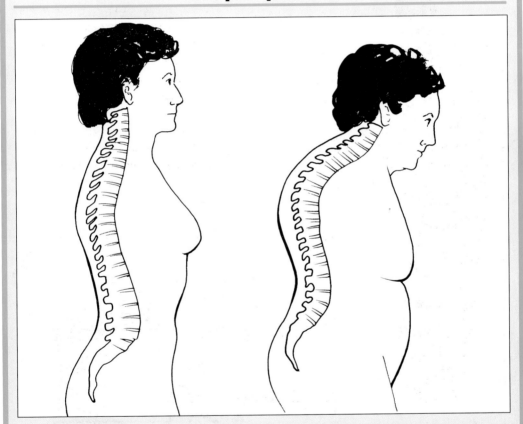

These illustrations show a normal spine (left) and an osteoporotic spine (right). Osteoporosis related fractures do heal but the bones do not go back to their original shape. The healed fractures become compressed or may mend in a wedge shape. Multiple fractures of the spine can result in stooped posture, a loss of height and pain.

Your skeleton

Testing for early diagnosis

The largest study to be conducted on the effect of osteoporosis in women is underway in the United States and involves 6,000 women. It is called the Fracture Intervention Trial (FIT) and will seek to provide a definitive answer to the relationship between bone mass density and the rate of fractures.

Various tests can be conducted to identify women with increased bone turnover and bone loss. These tests include the measurements of biochemical indicators or 'markers' in the blood and urine. They can indicate whether someone is losing bone faster than it is being replaced. Such tests are valuable indicators of whether someone is at risk of developing porous bones even although they may still be heavy and strong at the time of testing. They can act as a warning.

Coupled with actual measurements of bone density, the tests provide a picture of the present state of play, plus a forecast of what the future may be likely to hold if progression is allowed to continue unchecked. Machines called DEXA, (Dual Energy X-ray Absorptio-meters) which employ an X-ray tube have become the standard means of measuring bone mass and are being used to detect those with low bone mass at the menopause. The machines seem expensive, but in reality, this is a small cost compared to the potential benefits and savings in the future. However, there are still many major hospitals which do not have one, and many women who could benefit from a DEXA test are being denied the opportunity to have one.

In the UK, the National Osteoporosis Society is now campaigning for every major hospital to have such a machine as a means to early diagnosis of osteoporosis, particularly at the time of the menopause.

Bone density measurements using ultrasound are much cheaper and have the advantage of not using radiation, but they are only practical for measuring knee caps and heel bones which rarely suffer from osteoporotic fractures. This limits their usefulness.

Bone density testing in the United States

Where DEXA services are available, about one in ten of those scanned have some underlying cause of osteoporosis such as hyperthyroidism or have a bone disease other than osteoporosis. The results have to be carefully and professionally interpreted if opportunities for other therapeutic treatments are not to be missed. In the United States, some big stores offer bone scans, and osteoporosis specialists there are deeply critical of the practice. There is far more to interpreting the results than getting a bone mineral density printout.

Hopefully, they will not take off in Britain, but developments in the United States often cross the Atlantic, sooner or later.

Genetics

So how much of our bone health depends on nature and the genetic inheritance from our parents, and how much is down to nurture? Dr Ashok Bhalla of the Royal National Hospital in Bath, told a recent conference hosted in London by the National Dairy Council how identical twins have some differences in the quality of their bones, even though they were genetically identical. Non-identical twins showed greater variation. He stated that: 'Eighty per cent of adult peak bone mass is governed by the genes. That still leaves 20 per cent that is governed by the environment.'

Wherever we start from, there is always room for improvement.

Other causes of osteoporosis

Before treatment, the doctor will check that your osteoporosis is not caused by another underlying problem. Osteoporosis can be associated with the following:

● Long-term or high-dose corticosteroid use – sometimes prescribed for asthma or rheumatoid arthritis. Corticosteroid therapy can be very successful in treating these problems but has an adverse effect on the bones.

● Overactive thyroid or too high a dose of thyroid hormone replacement.

● Hyperparathyroidism, in which the parathyroid glands are overactive, leading to excessive loss of bone.

● Cancer, especially myeloma.

● Lack of mobility.

● Rare inherited conditions such as Osteogenesis Imperfecta.

● Anorexia nervosa or overdieting.

● Bulimia (related to anorexia – excessive fasting, coupled with gorging and deliberate regurgitation of food).

● Maladsorption problems such as chronic liver disease and after gastrectomy operations.

● Hypogonadism in which male or female sex organs have not developed properly, resulting in low levels of male or female hormones.

Chapter three

Who is at risk?

Any of us could be at risk of developing osteoporosis at some time in our lives, and the older we become, the greater is the likelihoodof suffering from this debilitating condition. It is largely an affliction of old age, for which the foundations are laid earlier in life, through our genes and lifestyle. As we have already seen, a healthy diet, which contains adequate calcium, and exercise to build strong bones are extremely important in its prevention.

Risk factors

The risk factors include the following:

● Being female.

● Being over 50.

● Having an early menopause.

● Having a hysterectomy, particularly if the type of operation involves removing one or both ovaries.

● Women whose mother had osteoporosis.

● A chronic low intake of calcium in the diet.

● Insufficient exposure to sunshine.

● Being over-thin, although being overweight should not be seen as a means of avoidance.

● Anorexia nervosa, and bulimia, the slimmer's diseases.

● Women who have had lots of missed periods.

● Low levels of exercise.

● Chronic liver, kidney, and digestive diseases.

● Patients receiving corticosteroid treatment.

● Excessive exercise to a degree which stops menstruation from occurring.

● Smoking.

● Excessive consumption of alcohol.

● Not being of black African descent. Caucasians, Orientals and Asians are in the risk groups.

● Men or women who have lost several inches in height.

Vitamin D and sunshine

Rickets, the deficiency disease in which lack of vitamin D upsets the calcium and phosphorus metabolism is a disease of infants and small children which interferes with the proper development of bone. Vitamin D is obtained from a suitable diet and is also produced by the body itself through the action of sunlight on the skin.

It is known as the sunshine vitamin, and exposure to sunshine during the warm summer months is an essential ingredient in bone health. Vitamin D is a vital factor in the laying down of bone by the body.

Fair skinned people are adapted to make the best use of the sunshine available in Northern climates where the sun's rays are relatively weak. It is beginning to be a matter of concern that people with darker skins living in Britain may be falling short on their sunshine needs because the pigmentation of their skin acts as a barrier.

For anyone living in a cold climate, it is advisable to seek out the sun during the summer months because of the shortfall during winter. It is a matter of balance and obviously you should not overdo sunbathing and become burned. Excessive exposure to sun is a well-known risk factor for skin cancer, but health experts are becoming concerned that some people may be taking the anti-cancer message too far by excessive avoidance of the sun and the use of total sun-block creams.

Sunbathing is beneficial as a source of vitamin D, which is important for laying down bone in the body. As too much sun can damage the skin and has been linked to skin cancer, you should use a sunscreen.

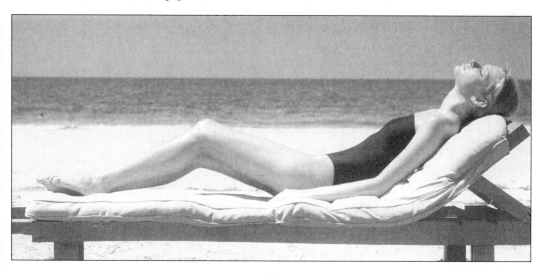

Who is at risk?

Anorexia

Anorexia nervosa, the disease in which sufferers who are usually female, but sometimes male, become locked in a pattern of excessive slimming, leads to deterioration of the bones. Even though other people can see that they are painfully thin and on a path that could lead to starving to death, the anorexic's own view is that they are still too fat and must plough on. When their monthly periods waver and halt as their body reacts to the shortage of food, the women's ovaries stop providing the hormones necessary for bone health. In effect, they are women who have become old before their time, with a premature menopause. There is a progressive loss of bone mass and although normal bone replacement will re-start after the anorexia has been overcome, the state of the bones will have suffered from the episode. From every aspect, a rapid return to normal eating patterns is desirable, as the longer the anorexic period continues, the greater will be the bone depletion.

Marathon risk

While exercise is an essential ingredient to good bone health, it is possible to have too much of a good thing. Some women marathon runners stop menstruating because of the over-harsh punishment their bodies are receiving. This invites bone decline because the working of their ovaries has been interrupted. Their periods will come back eventually when they moderate their level of exercise, but, like the anorexics, their bone density never returns to where it should have been. The extent of the damage depends on the length of time their periods have been absent. If rapid action is taken, little damage will have been done.

Women marathon runners who run many miles each week are among the high-risk groups for developing osteoporosis if they stop menstruating.

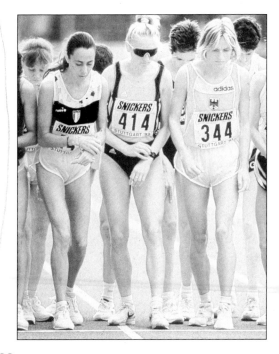

Smoking

The mechanism by which smoking affects the bones has not been explained. There are several hundred different chemical substances in tobacco smoke, and the main reasons for quitting smoking are to limit the risks of lung cancer and cardiovascular disease. It may be that substances in the smoke have a direct impact on the bones, or that the often poor diets of smokers play a contributory role. There is some evidence that women smokers may have an earlier menopause than non-smokers.

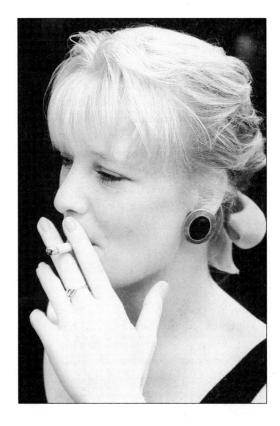

There are many reasons for giving up smoking, which is extremely damaging to health. Women who smoke have an increased risk of developing osteoporosis.

Alcohol

Alcohol only becomes a menace to the bones when drunk to excess. People who have an alcohol problem also tend to have notoriously deficient diets, and there are many other reasons why excessive drinking is harmful. The general health message is that women should not exceed 14 units of alcohol a week. A unit is the equivalent of a single measure of spirits, a glass of wine or half a pint of beer or lager. For men, the safe drinking limit is 21 units of alcohol a week. This way, we can enjoy drinking sensibly and stay healthy. People who drink excessively risk developing osteoporosis

Chapter four

The menopause

The National Osteoporosis Society is urging all UK women entering the menopause to consult their family doctor, even if they are not suffering the night sweats and hot flushes which make so many women's lives a misery during this period of change.

If you are entering your mid-life change your should expect to see the doctor, just as you expected to see a doctor when you were pregnant.

The majority of British women go through the menopause – change of life – without even realising that they should be seen and considered for hormone replacement therapy (HRT). Too often, women feel that they do not want to bother the doctor. However, there are many progressive doctors who feel that they should be bothered, and the medical profession is being encouraged to set up mid-life clinics, where women are provided with literature on osteoporosis and are given the opportunity to discover individually whether they are at risk and should be helped.

Examination may show good bone status and slow bone loss. If so, this is a bonus. But you should be given the opportunity to find out where you stand and what your own future is likely to hold. This is the best time to take positive action against any future crumbling of the bones, and heart disease too, which comes in the train of the menopause when the body is no longer making its own oestrogen hormone.

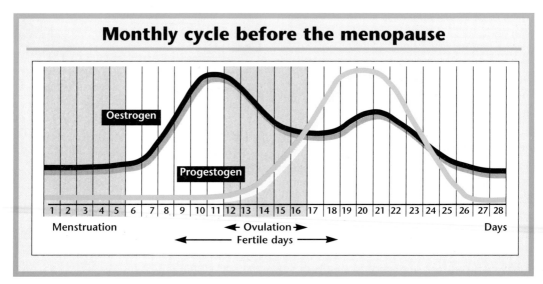

Monthly cycle before the menopause

Oestrogen

Progestogen

1 2 3 4 5 6 7 8 9 10 11 12 13 14 15 16 17 18 19 20 21 22 23 24 25 26 27 28

Menstruation   ◄ Ovulation ►   Days

◄——— Fertile days ———►

The menopause

This is the name given to the time in a woman's life when she stops having monthly periods and becomes unable to have any more children. It usually happens at around the age of 51 years, although some women can enter a premature menopause in their 30s, while others do not enter it until they are 55 or 56 years.

Smoking can bring on the menopause slightly earlier, but there is nothing that most women can do to alter the timing. The later the menopause, the greater is the advantage to the bones because they have enjoyed a longer period of natural protection and start the accelerated period of bone loss that much later.

The onset of menopause

Before the menopause the ovaries start to cut down on the production of oestrogen. Periods become less regular and eventually stop altogether. The release of eggs by the ovaries ceases. A premature menopause may occur naturally or if a woman's ovaries have been removed in an operation called oopherectomy. Women who have had their womb removed in a hysterectomy may also enter an early menopause. Women who undergo the menopause before the age of 50 may even lose half their bone stock by the time they reach their seventies. Experiencing the menopause later on brings added protection and delays the onset of bone loss.

The menopause is often a welcome relief not to have periods any more and also to get away from the monthly problem of premenstrual tension. However, it can be accompanied by unpleasant symptoms which may start many years before the last

Menopause symptons

- Hot flushes.
- Vaginal dryness.
- Thin and dry skin.
- Sleeping disturbances.
- Headaches.
- Night sweats.
- Depression.
- Irritability.
- Memory lapses.
- Fearfulness.
- Bladder infections.
- Stress incontinence (leaking urine).
- Sex becomes less enjoyable.
- A general feeling of being unable to cope and a loss of self-confidence.

The menopause

menstrual period and are due to a decline in oestrogen levels.

The list of symptons is not an attractive catalogue and women who used to feel that they were full of energy and in control of their lives, can feel they are losing their grip and that old age has arrived with a sickening suddenness. Problems with sleeping may mean they are tired during the daytime. Career women who feel their jobs are being put on the line are often more inclined to seek help than women who have stayed at home and have seen their families grow up and leave. But after raising a family, they deserve better than to be cast adrift into a situation where their ability to cope and to enjoy their new freedom to follow their own pursuits is being so severely hampered.

The menopause should not be dismissed as something that does not require any treatment. About three-quarters of women will be affected to some extent by one or more of the above symptoms. About a third

Menopause checklist

- Talk to your doctor and see if you could benefit from taking HRT.
- If you are experiencing unpleasant symptons, don't be afraid to ask your doctor for help and advice .
- Make sure that you are getting sufficient calcium in your diet.
- Try to exercise regularly – at least three times a week for 20 minutes.

find it is seriously interfering with the quality of their lives.

Although immediately debilitating, the symptoms do not have the disastrous long-term consequences of the insidious effects of bone depletion through lack of oestrogen and the lack of protection against coronary heart disease. These are the unseen disablers and killers which require just as much consideration as the more obvious symptoms.

Hormone replacement therapy

Deciding whether to go on to hormone replacement therapy (HRT) is not just a matter of feeling unwell at the time of the decision. It can be an investment for the future in which the payoff is good health in years to come, even if you appear to be passing through the menopause without a hitch.

For those who do go on to HRT, after a few weeks there is a feeling of rejuvenation as the more unpleasant symptoms of the

menopause wane, and the clock seems to have been put back. Sex lives improve and women feel their vigour and zest for life return. Friends say they look younger, but this may be more a reaction to their new-found energetic attitude. Women who have made it public that they are on HRT include British MP Teresa Gorman, who became an active campaigner after aching joints triggered by the menopause rendered her incapable of even cutting a slice of bread. A negative association between the onset of rheumatoid arthritis and the use of non-contraceptive hormones has been reported in one study. Now, on HRT, Mrs Gorman describes herself as a 'recycled example of the feminine species'. She shocked the House of Commons by uttering the 'M word' – menopause – when she made it part of her political role to campaign for other women. Male colleagues were outraged, but now she finds them coming up to ask how their wives can be helped. Former Prime Minister Lady Thatcher and actresses Kate O'Mara and Joan Collins are all on HRT.

Protection against coronary heart disease

Most people hate the idea of taking any medication long term, but the major bonuses of taking oestrogen replacement are reaped through the long-term approach. The therapy restores the hormone status to which our bodies have been accustomed since the start of monthly periods.

Hormone replacement therapy continued for many years will reduce the relative risk of hip fractures in women to half or even less. Those who are put on HRT have the dual benefits of protecting their bones as well as receiving protection against coronary heart disease through medication with similar hormones to those which their bodies used to produce naturally during their earlier years. A woman who is considered not to be at risk of osteoporosis at the time of her screening, should still be told of the beneficial effects

against coronary heart disease, even if there are no other positive indicators.

Coronary heart disease is now the biggest single cause of death in the UK in post-menopausal women, and oestrogen replacement is probably the single most effective way of preventing it.

Bone loss

The latest official figures in the UK show that only £61 million is being spent on HRT each year, yet treating the broken bones and other problems caused by osteoporosis costs the Health Service more than £1 billion a year.

When oestrogen replacement is stopped, the rate of bone loss is resumed, but from a higher starting point. But if the woman is comfortable with HRT, there seems to be no reason why it should not be continued for life. There is some evidence that the life expectancy can be increased by three years.

A recent study published in the *New England Journal of Medicine* concluded, however, that at least seven years of oestrogen therapy is necessary to have a persistent long-term effect on bone density. It is also possible, the authors said, that post-menopausal women may be able to reverse some of their bone loss or prevent further bone loss even if they begin oestrogen therapy later in life.

Of those who are given a prescription for HRT, many do not take it to the pharmacy to get the pills or patches, indicating that more time should have been taken in explaining the benefits. There is also a rapid fall-off among those who do start on HRT and this is assumed to be partly caused by the

The menopause

resumption of monthly bleeding at a time when they would prefer to see the end of periods. But it should be appreciated that the major benefits are achieved by regarding it as a long-term therapy, which means not just taking it for weeks, but for years.

HRT and cancer

Cancer scares have deterred many women from adopting HRT, and taking oestrogen replacement long term has been linked with an increased risk of endometrial cancer – cancer of the lining of the womb. This is why most preparations, designed for women who still have wombs, now include the hormone progesterone to counter this risk. The monthly calendar packs provide a combination of oestrogen/progesterone for a number of days and straight oestrogen for the rest. Adding the progesterone helps the womb to cleanse itself by promoting monthly bleeds, similar to a period. This reduces the risk of endometrial cancer to below normal. HRT, therefore, acts as a protection against endometrial cancer.

Women who do not have a womb take oestrogen-only preparations because, without a womb, they cannot develop cancer at this site. In the UK, they are not subject to the dual prescription charge.

HRT and breast cancer

Breast cancer in relation to HRT is still a continuing area of research. With one in twelve women developing breast cancer at some time in their lives, it is inevitable that a number who are on HRT will develop breast cancer. A study carried out in Oxford of 4,500 British women taking HRT concluded that the risk of this type of cancer was not increased if HRT was taken for less than ten years. There is evidence of a small increase in the diagnosis of breast cancer after ten years of HRT, but no evidence of an increase in death. It has been suggested that the HRT group of women tend to be more meticulous about having regular check-ups, so that it is being detected at an earlier stage when the cancer can be best treated. What matters, though, is your own personal risk, whatever it is, and that will not change through taking HRT for five and probably ten years. In the intervening time, we will, through ongoing

When to start HRT

It is most beneficial to start taking HRT at or just after the menopause. This will not only help alleviate some symptons but it will also give protection against bone loss and help prevent osteoporosis. However, it can be also taken by older women either to treat or prevent osteoporosis.

Advantages of HRT

Medical evidence suggests that taking HRT can bring many benefits, including:
- It relieves menopause symptons, especially hot flushes, night sweats, tiredness, irritability, nervous tension.
- It helps reduce the risk of fractures if taken for at least five years, starting soon after menopause.
- It helps halt bone loss in osteoporosis sufferers.
- It may help reduce the risk of coronary heart disease.

Disadvantages of HRT

There are certain side-effects associated with taking HRT which you may experience. These include:
- Nausea – this is usually temporary.
- Breast tenderness – this usually disappears.
- Fluid retention with slight weight gain and swollen ankles.

Note: These side effects may be reduced by adjusting the dose of HRT or switching to a different type – ask your doctor for advice.

studies, know much more about whether there really is a link with breast cancer and, if so, to what extent it exists. Overall, the risks of taking HRT are relatively few compared to the benefits it can bring to your health and well-being.

HRT and smoking

It is a misconception to think that smokers, women with existing coronary heart disease and high cholesterol levels cannot take HRT. Along with women who do not have these problems, it conveys a measure of protection against coronary heart disease and can thus be of great benefit.

How long should you take HRT?

If HRT is well tolerated, there seems to be no reason why it should be stopped, even in your seventies or older. The oestrogen intervention rapidly stops bone loss at almost any age in menopausal women. There is a minority of women who cannot tolerate oestrogen because it gives them headaches and makes them feel depressed. Some have initial nausea and breast tenderness, but this soon fades. Others have to give up wearing skin patches if they develop a skin irritation from the action of the adhesive plaster on the skin. If this happens, they may be happier switching to pills.

Of even greater long-term concern than the obvious symptoms of the menopause, is the effect it has on the risk of osteoporosis and coronary heart disease. Prior to having the menopause, women are protected from coronary heart disease by their female hormones. As a general rule, it is men who

The menopause

suffer early from coronary heart disease, but after the menopause, women catch up and enter the age of heart risk.

Women who go through the menopause before the age of 50 may have lost half their bone stock by their seventies, mainly due to the early menopause.

Each year doctors in the UK see more than 60,000 hip fractures, 50,000 wrist fractures, 40,000 spinal fractures and about 50,000 other fractures related to osteoporosis.

With fractures of the spine, some recent research has shown that only one in ten are being seen by doctors because those experiencing the fractures are suffering in silence, not appreciating what is causing them so much pain and discomfort. Most worrying is the rapid increase in the disease. There are more than five times as many fractures now as there were in the 1960s.

It now remains to be seen whether there will be a dramatic increase in the uptake of HRT. Doctors at a 1993 conference of the Health Council on Osteoporosis in Paris spoke of their concern that so few women are currently prepared to take HRT.

They acknowledge that new approaches may be needed to tackle osteoporosis which do not cause monthly bleeds. Drugs called bisphosphonates, currently being researched hold great promise but much more needs to be known about them. They are specific to osteoporosis and bone health and do not have the multiple beneficial effects of HRT.

Chapter five

Hysterectomy

For more than 1,000 British women a week, hysterectomy, the surgical removal of the womb, is performed to cure the problem of excessive menstrual bleeding when other methods of treatment have failed, and to remove fibroid tumours of the womb and womb cancer.

It is the end of any opportunity for conception and childbirth, and the operation requires careful counselling to counter the feelings that they have become somehow less of a woman now that part of their feminine structure has been taken away. Afterwards,

though, there is a sense of relief that an organ that was causing problems has been removed, and after a spell when even picking up a book may, in some rare cases, seem an enormous physical strain, their strength returns and life continues in better health without the womb which had ceased to be an asset.

The early forties is the average age for having a hysterectomy, and if not followed by hormone replacement therapy (HRT), these women, and particularly those who have had their ovaries removed, will be

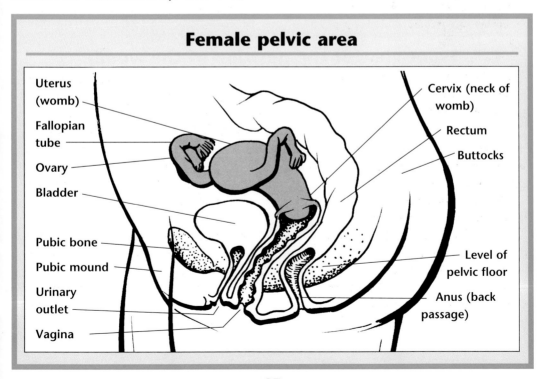

Female pelvic area

Uterus (womb)

Fallopian tube

Ovary

Bladder

Pubic bone

Pubic mound

Urinary outlet

Vagina

Cervix (neck of womb)

Rectum

Buttocks

Level of pelvic floor

Anus (back passage)

The menopause

plunged into an early menopause, with a vastly increased risk of developing future osteoporosis. The importance of long-term HRT cannot be too greatly emphasised.

As normally undertaken, the operation leaves a faint vertical or horizontal scar on the abdomen, necessitates 10 to 14 days in hospital, followed by a recovery period of six to eight weeks during which all heavy work should be avoided. The abdominal type of hysterectomy, which is performed through an opening in the abdominal wall, is the commonest type, and most surgeons aim to leave as little scarring as possible, with a thin scar along the bikini line so that there need be no embarrassment afterwards about wearing skimpy swimwear.

Some surgeons prefer to operate through the vagina (a vaginal hysterectomy), which leaves no external scars, but is not suitable for all conditions, and there may be good medical reasons why a scar-free operation is not always possible.

● **Total hysterectomies**, in which the whole uterus (womb) is removed, are more common. The word 'total' is misleading, because the ovaries are left in place. This is the usual type of operation for fibroids, prolapse or period problems which cause heavy and sometimes prolonged blood loss. For a period problem, a scrape is usually the first course of action and if this has failed to produce the desired result, a total hysterectomy may be indicated. As the cervix has been removed, smear tests are no longer needed by the woman.

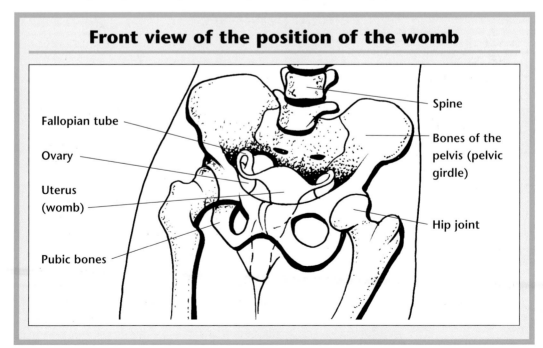

Front view of the position of the womb

Fallopian tube

Ovary

Uterus (womb)

Pubic bones

Spine

Bones of the pelvis (pelvic girdle)

Hip joint

● **Total hysterectomy with bilateral salpingo-oophorectomy** is the medical term for removing the womb, cervix, fallopian tubes and the ovaries. This operation is often the choice for women who have passed through the menopause or are over 50 years of age and whose ovaries are no longer active. It is conducted when there are large fibroids, cancer, long-standing pelvic infection or endometriosis – a painful condition of the lining of the womb. When it is conducted in premenopausal women, hormone replacement therapy is prescribed at the hospital, but too often those having the operation take their 'hospital pills' and then lapse, possibly because it has not been impressed with sufficient explanation that when the course has run out, they must continue with HRT through medication prescribed by their doctor.

● **'Extended' or 'Radical' or Wertheim's hysterectomy** are different terms describing the type of operation in which the womb, fallopian tubes, ovaries, cervix and the top of the vagina are removed, together with the surrounding fatty tissues and lymph glands in the pelvis. This is an extensive operation and is lusually performed for early cancer of the cervix, or of the endometrium – lining of the womb – in which the aim is to remove any local spread of the cancer. When the problem is discovered early in pre-cancer of the cervix, this can be cleared up by heat or laser treatment of the neck of the womb, thereby avoiding the need for surgery.

● **'Pelvic clearance'** is the term which is sometimes used as shorthand to describe a total hysterectomy with bilateral salpingo-oophorectomy or for extended or radical hysterectomy. Patients having any of these operations are not left with any empty space where their womb and other organs used to be. The bladder, bowel and intestines move around to take advantage of the extra room. The gap at the top end of the vagina, where the cervix used to be, is closed off by stitches. This may sound alarming, but in reality the womb is quite small (the size of a large pair) and the other organs will fill the space.

The uterus (womb)

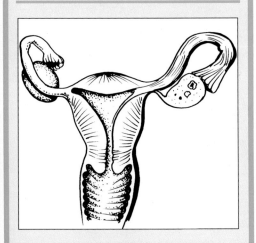

In total hysterectomy with bilateral salpingo-oophorectomy, the womb, cervix, fallopian tubes and ovaries are all removed. This operation is more common in women over 50 than in younger women.

The menopause

Delaying menopause symptoms

Once the ovaries have been removed, the body stops making oestrogen and progesterone. If working ovaries are to be removed, you will certainly need hormone replacement therapy, and should discuss this with the gynaecologist well ahead of the operation. HRT is vital for women in their thirties or forties. Even if the ovaries are kept, HRT after the operation should still be considered, to prevent menopausal symptoms and later bone and heart problems. Although some natural hormones will still be produced, women not taking HRT will encounter the gradual onset of menopausal symptoms, sometimes within two years.

Unlike many other operations, it is often clouded by fear and misunderstandings and old wives' tales over what to expect. Women who dreaded having the operation and thus delayed it, hoping that their embarrassing problems of menstrual flooding would disappear, now tell their friends that it heralded the beginning of a new life.

Types of hysterectomy operations

Total hysterectomy

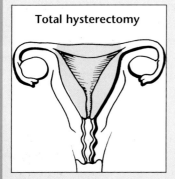

The whole womb is removed as shown, but the ovaries are left in place.

Total hysterectomy with bilateral salpingo-oophorectomy

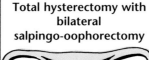
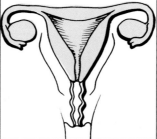

The womb, cervix, fallopian tubes and ovaries are removed.

'Extended' or 'Radical' Wertheim's hysterectomy

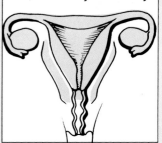

The womb, fallopian tubes, ovaries, cervix and the top of the vagina are removed.

Chapter six

Treatments

There are several treatments available for osteoporosis and the type selected by your doctor or specialist will depend, to some extent, on the severity of the symptoms and the underlying causes of the problem. Ideally, doctors will wish to have the results of a bone scan before engaging on a course of treatment. All treatments aim to provide pain relief, halt bone loss, prevent further fractures and replace or repair damaged bone.

Testosterone

Men are sometimes prescribed the male hormone testosterone to halt their osteoporosis, but they may need to be referred to a specialist centre for tests and treatment. Recent research has demonstrated a six per cent increase in bone density in men with osteoporosis of the spine who have been treated with testosterone for three years. These were men who had a deficiency of the hormone. The treatment has also been shown to increase bone density in some men with normal testosterone levels.

HRT

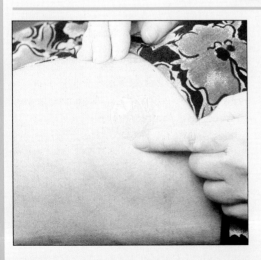

Hormone replacement therapy is the most likely treatment for women under 65 years of age, and can be carried out beyond this age. It is a safe and effective method of preventing further bone loss.For more details and information on HRT, turn to page 32.

Self-adhesive skin patches are impregnated with the female hormone oestrogen and release it into the skin. They are easy and painless to wear and an effective treatment in hormone replacement therapy.

Treatments

Calcitonin

Hormones called calcitonins are produced naturally by the thyroid gland and stop bone loss by blocking the action of the cells which break down bone. They are also found in certain fish where they regulate their adaption from sea water to fresh water. At specialist osteoporosis centres, consultants may prescribe calcitonin injections or a nasal spray or suppository as it cannot be given orally. Some synthetic versions of human calcitonin are available as well as synthetic salmon and eel calcitonins. Salmon calcitonins are the most commonly used.

The nasal sprays are not yet approved by the Medicines Control Agency in the UK for general prescription although they are widely available in continental Europe. Trials to date have shown nasal sprays and suppositories to be effective in halting bone loss, and side effects are less than with injections. A small number of people have said that they suffered from flushing, especially of the face and hands, and slight nausea.

One injectable type, Salcatonin, can be prescribed by doctors, but expense is a major drawback. Both men and women can be treated with calcitonins. Salmon calcitonin has a pain relieving action, which makes it suitable for the initial treatment of painful spinal osteoporosis, with drugs called bisphosphonates being substituted later in the course of the treatment.

Bisphosphonates

Bisphosphonates are chemical compounds which inhibit the loss of bone by sticking to the bone surface and thereby reducing the effectiveness of the cells which break down and destroy bone. The bisphosphonate etidronate has been widely prescribed in the UK for more than ten years for another bone condition called Paget's disease, and is now also prescribed for spinal osteoporosis in men and women. Studies have shown that it may reduce the number of fractures in the spine as well as halting bone loss. Little evidence has been collected as yet that it protects against hip fractures.

Etidronate in the form of Didronel PMO is taken for 14 days followed by a calcium supplement (Cacit) for 76 days. This cycle is repeated and continued for at least three years, and possibly indefinitely. The tablets should be taken with water or juice, two hours before or after food; otherwise it will not be adequately absorbed. It must not be taken with a milky drink, or coffee or tea, if they contain milk, because this will prevent the drug from being properly absorbed.

Side effects are rare, but if you do feel nauseous, this can be overcome by taking the etidronate at night. Mild diarrhoea is another rare side effect. Should the Cacit calcium supplement cause nausea or vomiting, ask your doctor to consider changing you to a different calcium supplement, but do not just stop taking the calcium.

Several other bisphosphonates are under investigationand are currently being tested. They may be simpler to take, and look extremely promising, and some specialists are already predicting they will be particularly useful to those older women who do not want to go on to HRT. These new drugs include alendronate, clodronate, pamidronate, risedronate and tiludronate.

Vitamin D

The family doctor may prescribe vitamin D on its own, or with etidronate, HRT, or calcium. Vitamin D acts as a bone strengthener by helping the body to absorb calcium. Vitamin D, the sunshine vitamin, is made naturally by your body, in response to the sun's rays, and is also obtained from foods such as cereals, milk, egg yolks and salt water fish. People who find it difficult to get out into the sunlight, may need vitamin supplements. There is a case for the over seventies taking calcium and vitamin D supplements.

Professor Pierre Meunier of the Hospital Edouard Herrot in Lyon, France, has reported that major benefits from supplementation were revealed by a study of 3,270 women living in homes for the elderly. The women who received a daily dose of 1,200 mg of calcium and 800 units of vitamin D3 had a 25 per cent reduction in the number of fractures after three years of treatment compared to those women who were not receiving the calcium and vitamin D supplements.

Anabolic steroids

Anabolic steroids which build up bone and muscle can be used to treat men with osteoporosis. However, they will masculinize women if used for three years or more, and sometimes sooner. Developing a moustache and a deeper voice are among the unwanted side effects which limit their use. They may also increase the risk of heart disease and liver problems. They can, though, be helpful in the very elderly, particularly if they are underweight and frail, and after a vertebral fracture. They have to be used with great caution and require careful monitoring.

Nandralone decanoate is the only anabolic steroid which is currently licensed for treatment of osteoporosis and this is given by injection once every two or three weeks. It appears to have a good pain relieving effect on the aching spines of many osteoporosis suffers.

Treatments

Fluoride

Sodium fluoride is occasionally used in small doses to restore bone density, and to reduce spinal fractures, but larger doses have an adverse effect on the bones and may actually increase the risk of a hip fracture. There is a very narrow margin of safety, and most specialists are now wary of using it. Those who do use it need to monitor progress carefully. It must be used with calcium supplements and it should only be prescribed by a specialist. Nausea, vomiting, diarrhoea and pains in the legs are sometimes reported as side effects.

Calcium

Calcium should be regarded as a nutrient rather than a medicine. A calcium-rich diet is helpful to the bones, but on its own will not stop osteoporosis. Calcium supplements can be beneficial to people with established osteoporosis, possibly combined with vitamin D supplements when the patient is very elderly or housebound.

Pain relief

There is no virtue in suffering in pain, when painkillers can reduce the discomfort. However, you must take special care never to exceed the recommended dose. Many people suffer severe pain, particularly if their spine has become weakened and more curved or fractured, whereas others suffer little or no pain.

Heat and cold

Heat pads, hot water bottles or ice packs may provide extra relief and it is worth experimenting to discover what helps. Put a cover on the hot water bottle to avoid burning.

Physiotherapy and other therapies

Physiotherapy and hydrotherapy are of great help to some osteoporosis patients, and acupuncture is helpful in some cases.

Some specialist centres now have Transcutaneous Electrical Nerve Stimulators (TENS) which can be strapped on to the painful area to block the pain messages from reaching the brain.

Tips for the elderly

It may sound like a statement of the very obvious, but for an elderly person to fracture a wrist or a hip, he or she has usually to fall.

Some people's bones are so brittle that they can be broken by an enthusiastic hug or a door slamming on them, but falls are the cause of most breakages.

Reducing accidents

While accidents do happen, much can be done to reduce the likelihood, and the home is the place where most accidents occur. This means conducting a thorough check to ensure that danger points such as curled and frayed carpet edges are remedied. Check the home for trailing flexes and poorly lit steps. The addition of a hand rail on the wall side of the stairs may be a useful safety measure. Many people who are familiar with their own homes, which they have lived in for years, think they know the layout so well that they can save electricity by not switching on extra lights. This is a false economy, and has resulted in many serious accidents. Loose rugs on highly polished floors can be another source of danger. Carpets give a softer landing if you do fall.

Ceramic floor tiles look elegant, but softer floor coverings with a better grip can be safer. Floorings which turn into skating rinks when newly swabbed, and provide a hard landing, can result in broken bones.

We become so familiar with our own homes that we often fail to see their potential pitfalls. A second opinion may be helpful in spotting the dangers that we ourselves fail to notice.

An American study comparing women who fell without fracturing a hip or wrist with others who fractured a hip, found that those who sustained a fracture tended to be taller or weighed more. Those who landed on a hard surface had a three-fold risk of hip fracture compared to those who fell on padded carpets, grass or unpaved dirt paths.

Nursing homes and homes for the elderly in the United States have found that the wearing of protective hip pads can be very effective in reducing the risk of hip fractures, even though they do not affect the risk of falling.

Exercise, even 20 minutes of walking, three times a week, can help people avoid falls by improving their balance and co-ordination. When we are young and quicker in our reactions, we are swifter at putting out an arm to break our fall. This can result in a broken arm or wrist, which can have its own serious consequences, but the damage is rarely as disabling as fracturing a hip. Any action which helps to break the fall reduces the energy being transmitted in the final impact, but as we grow older, we are less nimble at saving ourselves.

Continued on page 46

Treatments

Tips for the elderly

Continued from page 45
Falling sideways on to a hip is the worst way to fall. In judo, one of the first lessons is in how to break a fall by throwing out an arm so that the impact is spread evenly along the forearm from hand to elbow, with the full length of the forearm making contact. In judo, you also have a shock-absorbent padded mat to land on!

If you do find yourself falling, forget the shopping and handbag and give priority to saving yourself. It is more important to prevent broken bones than save half a dozen eggs from being smashed.

None of us likes to look as though we are getting less steady on our feet, but a four-wheel shopping trolley can act as a splendid walking frame while we are out and about, and people of all ages use them. A walking stick or a long, sturdy umbrella can be a valuable prop.

If you are unsteady on your feet and it is icy outside, there is no shame in accepting help from younger neighbours in doing some shopping for you.

Clothing

Clothes can be a problem if your spine is badly curved. However you can still look smart and attractive, and need not go in for dowdy dressing, which can be very depressing. If the neck gapes at the back, this may be improved by putting small darts on either side of the centre back, or, if there is a centre back seam, shaping it into the neck. An attractive scarf draped over the shoulders can look like a fashion accessory, while hiding any defects.

If your tummy has bulged as a result of osteoporosis, and the hems ride up and dip, levelling the hem line can make a big difference. Blouses and skirts may be easier to manage than dresses. If the blouse is not tucked in, it can cover a bulging tummy, but do not try to pull yourself in with tight corsets. Garments with side zips or front buttons may be easier to take on and off than ones with zips at the back.

The National Osteoporosis Society has produced an excellent guide, 'Straighten up with Fashion', which was written with help from the London College of Fashion to give useful tips and advice on clothing problems to osteoporosis sufferers.

Lifetime plan
Sufficient calcium in the diet, and exercise, should be the mainstay of our lifetime plan from youth to old age.
Birth to aged 20
Adequate calcium in the diet and exercise.
20 to 50 years
Avoid risk factors.
50 to 70
Oestrogen and progestogen (HRT).
Aged 70 plus
Calcium and vitamin D supplement.

Make your home accident-safe

- Fit bath rails and a non-slip bath mat to make getting in and out of the bath easier.
- Consider installing a walk-in shower.
- Fit a hand rail no the stairs.

- Avoid rugs and frayed carpet edges.
- Take care on wet and slippery floors.
- Avoid trailing flexes and wires.

Keep staircases well lit.

Summary

Various treatments are available for treating osteoporosis and you must consult your doctor or specialist to find out what is best for you. However, you can help yourself by ensuring that you get sufficient calcium in your diet as well as adding vitamin D. These are not treatments in themselves but they may help to reduce fractures.

Chapter seven

Your diet

Our bones consist largely of calcium, and calciumwe derive from our diets is incorporated to provide them with their rigidity and strength.

We need calcium to build the bones in the first place and to maintain the strength of our skeletons. Cell by cell, children replace their entire skeletons once every two years because the old bone is constantly being removed and new bone put in its place, plus some additional bone as part of the growing process. Adults typically replace their entire skeleton every seven to ten years.

It is therefore important throughout life to ensure that the calcium intake is sufficient to develop and maintain a strong and very healthy skeleton. This is particularly important during childhood, through adolescence, whilewomen are pregnant and later on in old age.

Children's diets

Of current concern is the trend among children to consume so many fizzy drinks, whereas, formerly, they would have been drinking more milk. Slick advertising has made fizzy drinks fashionable, and children are no more immune to items they see advertised on television than are adults. Parents find it difficult to resist these pressures

UK surveys on children's diets

One UK survey of Welsh schoolchildren has shown that about 50 per cent are eating a diet that is calcium deficient. A scientifically controlled study of some identical twins has now confirmed the benefit of taking supplementary calcium in childhood.

A recent survey conducted for the British National Dairy Council found that of 220 children, around 11 per cent of boys and 23 per cent of girls over the age of five do not include enough milk and milk products in their diet for optimum bone growth. In children aged 5-11 years, 6 per cent of boys and 12 per cent of girls were not getting enough calcium. In the age group 11-18 years, 17 per cent of boys and 21 per cent of girls had calcium-deficient diets.

Calcium for children

You can ensure that your child gets sufficient calcium by:
- Eating breakfast cereal with milk
- Providing milky drinks, e.g. hot drinks, milkshakes
- Serving sardines or pilchards on white toast for tea or mashed in sandwiches
- Eating cheese or adding a cheese topping to soups and hot dishes
- Providing green vegetables with meals
- Adding seeds or nuts to dishes
- Serving yogurt as a dessert or snack food

when the children do not want to be the odd ones out and ask for the same products that their friends are drinking. Indeed, the whole spectrum of children's diets is being distorted towards crisps and snacks and away from healthy balanced meals. The calcium picture is only part of a much wider concern over the nutrition of growing children.

There may be a case for bringing back school milk, not for reasons of poverty, as was the case when it was first introduced, but to restore the dietary balance in an increasingly fashion-driven world.

Ideally, we should not need to feed any calcium supplements to our children if getting enough from their food is achievable.

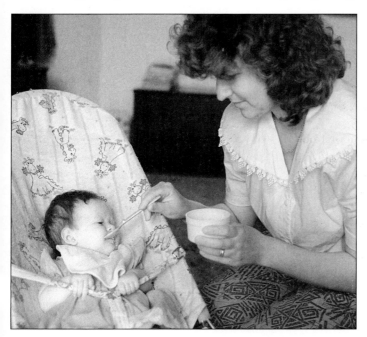

It is very important that children eat a varied, healthy diet in their formative years. Calcium is essential for building strong, healthy bones, and this can be supplied by such foods as milk, yogurt, cheese, green leafy vegetables and sardines. Try to ensure that your child gets sufficient milk each day.

Your diet

Eating a balanced diet

Doctors, nutritionists and dietitians all agree that a healthy balanced diet is necessary to supply the body with energy, essential nutrients, vitamins and minerals and fibre. A healthy diet contains a balanced amount of:

- Fruit and vegetables.
- Bread and cereals.
- Milk and dairy products.
- Lean meat, poultry, fish, eggs, nuts and pulses, such as beans.

We are eating less food than we used to in the past, yet we are growing fatter, which reflects the fact that we are getting less exercise than we used to and are not burning up as many calories through physical activities.

Figures from the British Ministry of Agriculture, Fisheries and Food (MAFF) reveal a decline in calcium intake over the past 30 years. Back in 1960, the average UK intake of calcium for men, women and children was 1,040 mg per day, but this has fallen steadily over the years to 817 mg per day in 1990.

Vitamin D

You need this to absorb the calcium in the food you eat. Apart from sunlight, you can get vitamin D from your daily diet by eating the following:

- Oily fish, eg. sardines, mackerel, herring
- Cod liver oil
- Milk and butter
- Egg yolk
- Foods that are fortified with vitamin D, e.g. breakfast cereals, skimmed milk powder, margarine

The decline in total calcium intake can be attributed largely to the decreased consumption of milk and, to a lesser extent, white bread. Although there has been an upsurge in the purchase of reduced-fat milks and a small increase in cheese consumption,

Children who don't like milk or cheese

You can ensure that your child eats calcium-rich foods even if he doesn't like milk or cheese

- Mix milk and yogurt or milk powder into soups and sauces.
- Make your own ice-creams and mousses with milk.

- Mix yogurt into fruit purées.
- Mix low-fat soft cheese into mashed vegetables.
- Sprinkle mild cheese onto vegetables and stews and grill until crisp and golden.
- Make hot, milky drinks.
- Whizz up a fruit milk shake.

this has not compensated for the fall in total milk consumption.

A UK joint survey by the Office of Population Censuses and Surveys, MAFF and the Department of Health of British adults published in 1990 showed that average daily calcium intakes for men were 940 mg and 730 mg for women. But the younger age groups tended to be getting smaller amounts of calcium. The intake of those aged 16-24 was significantly lower than those aged 35-64.

Although calcium intakes of most adults would appear to be adequate, those of some children give cause for concern. Results of a Department of Health survey published in 1989 showed that average calcium intake for boys was 833 mg per day at age 10-11, rising to 925 mg per day at 14-15 years. For girls, average values were lower and fell from 702 mg per day at age 10-11 years to 692 mg per day at 14-15 years.

These levels are considerably lower than the current Reference Nutrient Intakes of 1,000 mg per day for boys and 800 mg per day for girls in this age group.

The best sources of calcium are milk, cheeses and yogurt which all contain high amounts and are easily absorbed by the body. Adults who are concerned to avoid furring the arteries by reducing the intake of dairy fat, can opt for low-fat milks, cheeses and yogurts. Low-fat products contain as high and sometimes higher levels of calcium than full-fat varieties. Adults watching their waistlines can switch to skimmed milk to maintain their calcium intake.

Recommended calcium intake in the UK

Age	Calcium Reference Nutrient Intake mg/day
1-3	350
4-6	450
7-10	550
11-18 male	1,000
11-18 female	800
19-50	700
50 plus	700
Pregnancy	700
Breastfeeding	1,250
Breastfeeding (under 19)	1,350

Vegetarians

Vegetarians who can eat and drink milk products should be able to maintain their calcium levels with ease. For vegans, who will eat nothing derived from animals, it is more difficult and requires a more studied approach if a shortfall is to be avoided. Nutritionists confess that there is a lack of knowledge about the nutritional status of children on vegan and other minority diets. So many dietary studies have been focused on obscure parts of the globe and it is a matter of concern that so little is known about what is happening in our own society.

Your diet

Increase your calcium consumption

Although some foods are very high in calcium, such as leafy green vegetables like spinach and broccoli fibre-rich foods and nuts, the calcium can be far less well absorbed than in dairy foods. Substances such as oxalates in vegetables and possibly components of dietary fibre in cereals, impair the absorption of calcium from the small intestine, reducing the amount that is actually available to the body.

● In the UK hite and brown bread is made from flour fortified with calcium, (under Bread and Flour Regulations of 1984), but not wholemeal flour, although some bread manufacturers add it during the bread-making process. Wholemeal bread is quite rich in calcium but the phatic acid it contains prevents its total absorption by the body.

● Canned fish, which contains fish bones in an edible form, is a good source of calcium, especially canned sardines and pilchards.
● Some nuts and seeds contribute substantial amounts of calcium, especially Brazil nuts and almonds, but only for people who eat them regularly.
● Drinking certain mineral waters and water from the tap in hard-water areas can provide about 220mg of calcium a day. However, tap water in soft-water areas provides virtually no calcium.
● Vegetables, especially green ones, are also a good source of calcium. Serve them with meals, cooked or in salads or as 'dippers' with a cheese or yogurt dip.
● You can also get calcium from some fruit, especially dried fruit such as figs, prunes and apricots.

Boost your calcium

It is thought that three-quarters of women get inadequate calcium in their daily diet – less than the 500mg minimum daily requirement. Pregnant women need twice this amount, whereas osteoporosis sufferers would benefit from three times as much.

The following quick checklist is of foods that contain approximately 300mg calcium:
● 50g/2oz hard cheese
● 250g/8 floz milk
● 200g/7oz yogurt
● 100g/4oz sardines or other fish with bones, e.g. whitebait
● 150g/5oz nuts, especially almonds and Brazil nuts

Typical calcium contents of some calcium-rich foods

Note: 28g is equivalent to 1oz

Weight (g)	Food	Calcium (mg)
	Dairy foods	
150g	Yogurt (low fat fruit	225
188ml	Skimmed milk	235
188ml	Semi-skimmed milk	231
188ml	Silver Top milk	224
28g	Cheddar cheese	202
28g	Edam cheese	216
28g	Cottage cheese plain	20
112g	Cheese and tomato pizza	235
112g	Ice cream, dairy	134
56g	Milk chocolate	123
56g	Mars Bar	90
	Fish	
56g	Whitebait, fried	482
56g	Salmon, canned	52
56g	Sardines canned in tomato sauce	258
56g	Pilchards canned in tomato sauce	168

Weight (g)	Food	Calcium (mg)
	Bread	
30g (1 slice)	White bread	33
30g (1 slice)	Wholemeal bread	16
	Vegetables	
112g	Spinach, boiled	179
112g	Broccoli, boiled	45
112g	Winter cabbage, boiled	43
112g	Spring greens, boiled	84
28g	Watercress	48
	Nuts and Seeds	
56g	Brazil nuts	95
56g	Hazelnuts	78
56g	Almonds	134
56g	Peanuts	33
14g	Sesame seeds	94
	Fruit	
28g	Dried figs	76
	1 large orange	58
112g	Baked beans, cooked	59
112g	Red kidney beans, cooked	80

Alternatives to milk

Commercial calcium-fortified soya milk can be bought by those who cannot, or do not wish to drink ordinary milk and there are calcium supplements available. A day's meals for someone on a Vegan diet could include steamed soya bean curd: 84g/3oz will provide 428mg of calcium. This amount of bean curd, together with 550ml/1 pint of soya milk, one portion of vegetable and bean casserole, 4 slices of bread, a portion of muesli, some dried figs and 84g peanuts will add up to almost 1,000mg of calcium.

Calcium boosting

Note: A pregnant teenager can get just over 1,500mg from drinking 550ml/1 pint semi-skimmed milk, and eating a portion of tomato with Caerphilly cheese, 2 slices of bread, a carton (150ml/5floz) low-fat fruit yogurt and a portion of spiced chicken with spinach.

Your diet

Calcium intake for the elderly

A daily intake of 1,500mg of calcium is recommended for sufferers from osteoporosis and the elderly. Elderly people absorb calcium and other minerals less efficiently and it is particularly important to maintain a good balanced diet in later life, and, if necessary, to take calcium and vitamin D supplements when 70 years or older. A pint of milk a day should be the aim, using it on cereals, in tea, custard, desserts, milky coffee and malted or chocolate drinks to give variety.

Recipes with calcium

Here is a selection of delicious recipes, provided by the National Osteoporosis Society, that will help you increase the calcium in your daily diet. They are all made with nutritious ingredients and can be included in a normal healthy, balanced eating plan. We have chosen recipes that are relatively high in calcium and have given you the calcium content and sources.

Cod and prawn florentine

450g/1lb fresh spinach
325g/12oz cod fillet, skinned
100g/4oz cooked, peeled prawns
15g/½oz butter
15g/½oz plain flour
300ml/½ pint milk
150g/5oz grated Cheddar cheese
salt and pepper
25g/1oz fresh breadcrumbs
tomato and parsley to garnish

1 Wash the spinach in cold water and remove the stalks. Cook, without adding any water, for 5 minutes. Drain and chop finely, and then transfer to an ovenproof dish.

2 Cut the cod into 2.5cm/1 inch cubes. Scatter the cod and prawns over the spinach.

3 Melt the butter in a small saucepan and stir in the flour to make a roux. Cook for a few minutes, then gradually blend in the milk. Bring to the boil, stirring continuously until the sauce thickens. Remove from the heat and stir in 100g/4oz of cheese.

4 Pour the cheese sauce over the fish. Mix together the remaining cheese and breadcrumbs and sprinkle over the top. Bake in a preheated oven at 200°C/400°F/Gas Mark 6 for 20 minutes. Garnish with sliced tomato and parsley.

Serves: 4

Calcium: 560mg per portion

Sources: prawns, cheese, milk, breadcrumbs, spinach

Chive and salmon pancakes

100g/4oz plain flour

¼ teaspoon salt

2 tablespoons chopped fresh chives

1 size-3 egg

300ml/½ pint milk

2 tablespoons oil

For the filling:

15g/½oz butter

2 sticks celery, sliced

225g/8oz curd cheese

2 tablespoons milk

1 small green pepper, chopped

200g/7oz can salmon

salt and freshly ground black pepper

4-5 tablespoons single cream

1 Make the pancakes: sift the flour and salt into a bowl, make a well in the centre and add the chives and egg. Beat with a wooden spoon, gradually adding the milk to form a smooth batter.

2 Heat a little of the oil in a small frying pan and pour in a little batter, tipping the pan so that it covers the base. Cook until the edges start to curl, then flip the pancake over and fry the other side until golden. Make all the pancakes in this way and keep them warm while you make the filling. This quantity of batter makes 8 pancakes.

3 To make the filling: melt the butter in a small saucepan and sauté the celery until soft. Put the curd cheese in a bowl and stir in the milk. Mix in the celery, green pepper, salmon and seasoning.

4 Divide the filling mixture between the pancakes and roll up. Arrange in an ovenproof dish and spoon the cream over the top. Bake in a preheated oven at 180°C/350°F/Gas Mark 4 for 15 minutes. Serve with warm granary rolls.

Serves: 4

Calcium: 380mg per portion with granary rolls

Sources: milk, curd cheese, salmon

Calcium cookery tips

1 Drink a glass of milk with your meals.
2 Stir some milk or yogurt into soups.
3 Choose calcium-rich vegetables, e.g. broccoli, beans.
4 Make yogurt-based salad dressings.
5 Serve a white sauce with fish or vegetables.
6 Sprinkle grated cheese over soups and pasta.
7 For between-meal snacks and nibbles, eat dried apricots, low-fat cheeses.
8 Use fruit-flavoured fromage frais as a topping for fruit and desserts.
9 Add grated cheese to savoury shortcrust pastry.
10 Make yogurt dips and serve with raw vegetables.
11 Top baked potatoes with yogurt and chives or grated cheese.
12 Make a quick milkshake by blending milk with fruit yogurt.

Your diet

Calcium at breakfast time

1 Start the day with a bowl of wholewheat cereal and milk. An average portion will provide 240mg calcium as well as protein, starch, fibre, minerals and vitamins.

2 A bowl of porridge is a warming breakfast for cold mornings. Make it with milk, not water, to boost the calcium content and serve with fruit, milk, sugar, or salt if you are traditionally minded. An average bowl contains about 200mg calcium.

3 French toast, or eggy bread, is another good source of calcium. Just beat together 2 eggs, 75g/3oz grated Cheddar cheese and 50ml/2 fl oz milk. Dip slices of white bread into this mixture, then fry in oil until crisp and golden on both sides. An average portion contains about 220mg calcium.

4 Yogurt is a quick and delicious way of increasing your calcium. Try a 150g/5oz pot plain low-fat yogurt served with a dried fruit compote for approximately 240mg calcium.

5 For a quick and refreshing breakfast drink, put 1 banana, 150ml/5 fl oz apricot yogurt and 150ml/5 fl oz milk in a blender with a few ice cubes. Blend until thick and frothy for 250mg calcium.

Pasta salad with lemon dressing

75g/3oz pasta spirals, cooked and cooled

100g/4oz Double Gloucester cheese, diced

200g/7oz can salmon

1/4 cucumber, sliced

50g/2oz sweetcorn kernels

For the dressing:

2 tablespoons oil

grated rind and juice of 1 lemon

1/4 teaspoon sugar

1/4 teaspoon mustard powder

salt and pepper

1 tablespoon chopped fresh parsley

1 Put the pasta spirals, cheese, salmon, cucumber and sweetcorn kernels in a large bowl and mix them gently together.

2 Place all the ingredients for the salad dressing in a screwtop jar and shake well until mixed.

3 Pour the dressing over the salad and toss lightly until all the ingredients are coated with dressing.

Serves: 2

Calcium: 490mg per portion

Sources: cheese, salmon

Broccoli and cauliflower bake

225g/8oz broccoli

225g/8oz cauliflower

25g/1oz butter

25g/1oz plain flour

300ml/$^1/_2$ pint milk

50g/2oz Caerphilly cheese, grated

salt and pepper

pinch of mustard powder

50g/2oz flaked almonds

1 Break the broccoli and cauliflower into florets and cook in boiling salted water for 5 minutes. Drain and place the vegtables in an ovenproof dish.

2 Melt the butter in a small saucepan and stir in the flour to make a roux. Cook over gentle heat for 2-3 minutes. Gradually add the milk, stirring continuously until the sauce boils and thickens. Remove from the heat and add the grated cheese. Stir until melted and then season the sauce with salt and pepper and mustard powder.

3 Pour the sauce over the broccoli and cauliflower, and sprinkle with the almonds. Bake in a preheated oven at 200°C/400°F/Gas Mark 6 for 30 minutes. Serve with baked potatoes.

Serves: 2

Calcium: 615mg per portion

Sources: milk, cheese, broccoli, almonds

Cheese and herb pudding

8-10 slices white bread, crusts removed

40g/1 $^1/_2$oz butter

100g/4oz mushrooms

100g/4oz Lancashire cheese, crumbled

3 size-3 eggs

550ml/1 pint milk

1 teaspoon mixed dried herbs

salt and pepper

1 Lightly butter the bread, and cut it into fingers or squares. Arrange a layer of buttered bread in the bottom of a greased ovenproof dish. Cover with a layer of mushrooms and then one of cheese. Continue layering up in this way, finishing with a layer of bread.

2 Beat together the eggs, milk, herbs, salt and pepper. Pour this mixture over the bread and set aside to stand for 30 minutes.

3 Bake the pudding in a preheated oven at 170°C/325°F/Gas Mark 3 for 1 hour, or until the egg mixture has set and the top is golden brown. Serve with fresh green beans.

Serves: 4

Calcium: 495mg per portion served with beans

Sources: bread, cheese, milk

Your diet

Beef and bean pie

350g/12oz lean minced beef

1 onion, finely chopped

450g/1lb can baked beans

215g/7 $^1/_2$oz can butter beans, drained

1 tablespoon tomato purée

dash of Worcestershire sauce

450g/1lb potatoes

25g/1oz butter

2 tablespoons milk

salt and pepper

50g/2oz Red Leicester cheese, grated

1 Cook the mince and onion in a saucepan
without adding any fat, until the beef is
browned. Drain off any fat.

2 Stir in the beans, tomato purée and
Worcestershire sauce. Bring to the boil and
simmer for 15 minutes.

3 While the mince is cooking, boil the
potatoes. When they are cooked, mash with
butter, milk and seasoning.

4 Transfer the mince to an ovenproof dish
and cover with the mashed potato. Fluff it up
with a fork and sprinkle with grated cheese.
Bake in a preheated oven at 180°C/350°F/Gas
Mark 4 for 25 minutes until the cheese is
bubbling and hot. Serve with broccoli.

Serves: 4

Calcium: 310mg per portion served with broccoli

Sources: cheese, baked beans, milk, broccoli

Surprise burgers

450g/1lb lean minced beef

1 onion, grated

50g/2oz fresh white breadcrumbs

1 teaspoon mixed dried herbs

salt and pepper

1 size-3 egg, beaten

100g/4oz grated Double Gloucester

1 Put all the ingredients, except the cheese,
in a large bowl and mix together well. Divide
the mixture into 4 equal-sized portions.

2 Shape each portion into a burger, putting a
quarter of the cheese in the centre of each.
Leave in a cool place for 30 minutes.

3 Cook the burgers under a preheated grill
for about 7 minutes each side. Serve with a
salad of shredded cabbage, grated carrot,
raisins and peanuts dressed with yogurt.

Serves: 4

Calcium: 300mg per portion with salad

Sources: cheese, breadcrumbs

How to get calcium

The best sources of calcium are as follows:
- Milk
- Yogurt
- Eggs
- Cheese
- Sardines
- Beans
- Leafy green
  vegetables

Cheese and broccoli quiche

175g/6oz plain flour

1/2 teaspoon salt

1/2 teaspoon mixed dried herbs

75g/3oz butter

For the filling:

15g/1/2oz butter

1 onion, chopped

225g/8oz broccoli, cut in small pieces

2 size-3 eggs

300ml/1/2 pint milk

100g/4oz grated Double Gloucester or Blue Stilton cheese

salt and pepper

1 Make the pastry: sift the flour and salt into a bowl, and mix in the herbs. Rub in the butter. Add enough cold water to make a firm dough.

2 Roll out the pastry and line a 20cm/8 inch flan ring. Prick the base with a fork, line with greaseproof paper and fill with baking beans. Bake 'blind' in a preheated oven at 200°C/400°F/Gas Mark 6 for 20 minutes.

3 Melt the butter and fry the onion until softened. Spread across the base of the pastry case, and arrange the broccoli on top.

4 Beat the eggs, milk, cheese and seasoning together. Pour over the broccoli. Bake at 200°C/400°F/Gas Mark 6 for 15 minutes, then reduce to 180°C/350°F/Gas Mark 4 for a further 20-30 minutes. Serve with a green salad.

Serves: 4

Calcium: 430g per portion served with green salad

Sources: cheese, milk, broccoli, flour

When you need extra calcium

● **Slimmers.** It is essential that slimmers following a low-fat diet do not cut out dairy products. They can get adequate calcium by choosing low-fat yogurt, cheeses, skimmed milk and green vegetables.

● **In pregnancy.** You need plenty of calcium in your diet to build your unborn baby's bones. If you do not eat enough calcium, the baby will rob your own supplies.

● **In childhood.** Children need calcium for building healthy bones. If they eat sufficient calcium, they are better equipped to withstand bone loss in later life.

● **In adolescence.** This is a peak time for bone development and teenagers need a high intake of calcium. During these years, 37 per cent of the adult skeleton is formed.

● **The elderly.** As you get older you absorb calcium less efficiently so it is essential to eat a calcium-rich diet, possibly with calcium supplements as well.

Chapter eight

Exercise

p 8

Exercise, building up gradually and never punishing yourself too hard, is an important part of the picture for keeping the bones healthy and strong.

Weight-bearing exercise is the best for bones, but that does not mean you need to go to the gymnasium to lift weights, although weight-training is certainly one way. Walking is the most easily available form of weight-bearing exercise, whether walking the dog, fell-walking, or walking a couple of stops more before catching the bus.

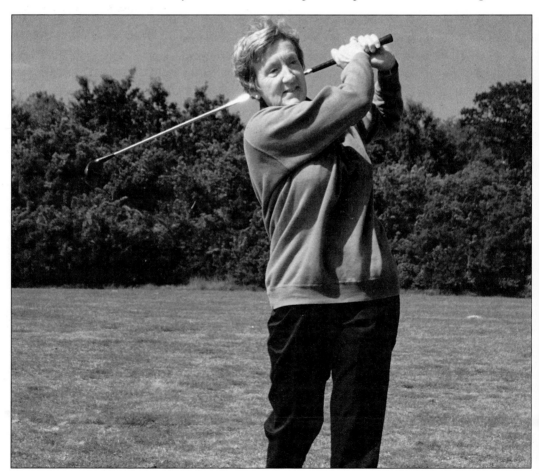

Think before climbing into the car whether the journey could be done just as well on foot. Golf is a splendid way of adding up the miles without making it seem like a chore. Any form of physical sports will do, but beware of plunging straight from being a couch potato onto the squash court, where over-exertion can be dangerous for those who are unfit. If you are unused to exercise your doctor may help you to plan out a suitable exercise programme.

It is a question of finding what suits you, whether it is walking, jogging, running, step aerobics or vigorous sports, and engaging in some form of exercise three times a week, or preferably on a daily basis. Dancing, playing tennis and 'keep fit' exercises are all good. Start off gently, if you are not used to it. Swimming is a good reintroduction to exercise. It improves mobility and can pave the way for taking weight-bearing exercise which is more helpful to the bones.

It is not known exactly how exercise alters bone, but in some way, the result of stressing the bones is to encourage the osteoblasts, the bone-building cells, to greater activity in creating new cells, and the bone demolition cells, the osteoclasts, may work more slowly, giving an overall gain in bone or slowing down the rate of bone loss.

Beneficial effects of exercise have been observed in younger people who have been

Golf is an enjoyable way of exercising as you have to walk several miles around an 18-hole course. You are never too young nor too old to play and it appeals to all ages.

unable to exercise during a spell of illness. When they start exercising again, the beneficial effects on the bones can be demonstrated within six months. In the over-seventies, it may take longer for the bones to respond.

In America, studies of women aged 30 to 40 found that groups starting regular weight-training showed an increase in bone mass. Runners did even better, but women from the same age group living a sedentary lifestyle continued to lose bone. Exercise is known to help build up bones, but it is not known whether the beneficial effects for older adults are lost when the exercise stops. There are, though, reasons to believe that if the exercise has to stop because of illness or some other problem, the skeleton starts from a position of greater strength, with 'more bone in the bank'.

No-one can give a precise recipe for the best types of exercise and how much.

Children

Researchers at the University of Exeter in the UK who monitored the activity of a group of schoolchildren for three successive days found that 87 per cent of girls and 76 per cent of boys did not reach any sustained periods of vigorous activity, and they did very little on Saturdays. Girls from the age of 12 onwards were particularly inactive. Children who play sport tend to be the ones who continue as adults, and physical educationalists are concerned that too few youngsters are setting the groundwork for good exercise habits. Curiously, the exercise habits of parents do not seem to be reflected

Exercise

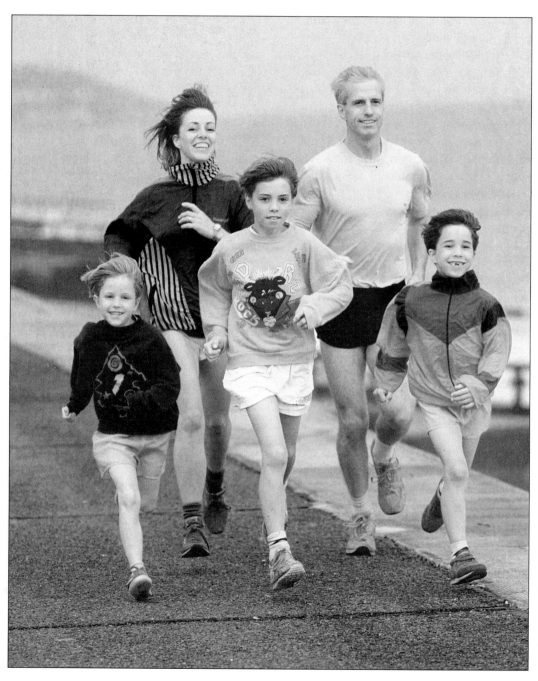

by their children in most cases, and having sporty parents is no guarantee that the children will follow suit.

It may be that too many children are being deterred if they do not have a natural talent for ball games, but the health message is about exercise and not about winning or scoring goals. We may need to do more to encourage youngsters who are not naturally sporty to put in more time in their local gymnasium working out, or to find a form of exercise that they enjoy which is non-competitive.

Athletes and dancers

At the other extreme are young female athletes and dancers, who have exercised beyond healthy limits and have seen their monthly cycle switch off. These are the ambitious elite athletes and dancers, and 30 to 50 per cent of such women are estimated to develop oestrogen deficiency, loss of periods and a predisposition to later osteoporosis.

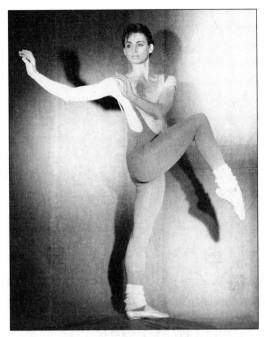

Dancers must take special care to get enough calcium in their daily diet. Professionals risk developing oestrogen deficiency and are at risk of getting osteoporosis later in life.

The elderly

The UK charity Age Concern is taking a lead in encouraging older members of our society to take healthy exercise, as part of 'Look After Yourself' courses. Organised exercise is a key part of their new Ageing Well project in which Age Concern has formed an alliance with drug company Merck Sharp &

It is a good idea to exercise together as a family, which will benefit both adults and children. You can go out jogging or cycling at weekends, or visit your local swimming pool or leisure centre.

Dohme, health insurers Private Patients Plan and the UK Department of Health to raise public awareness of healthy ageing. Nine projects in different parts of the country are laying the groundwork for the scheme to spread nationwide, with older volunteers being professionally trained to spread the health message. Some of the projects involve organised exercise classes for the over-fifties.

For people, usually elderly, who are already bowed and disabled by osteoporosis, referral to a physiotherapist can be of considerable help in restoring some mobility. The physiotherapist will help advise on

Exercise

Hydrotherapy exercises

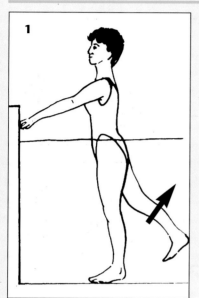

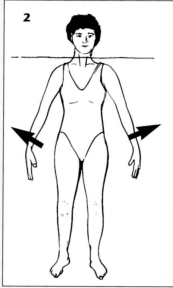

2 Resting your back against the side of the pool with arms out in front, stretch them back to the wall. Repeat 5 times.

1 Stand facing the edge of the pool, arm length away and touching it with your fingertips. Keeping the knee straight, raise and stretch one leg back behind you. Repeat with the other leg. Repeat 5 times with each leg.

3 Stand with arms floating up in front of you. Push them down into the water and back behind you. Repeat 5 times.

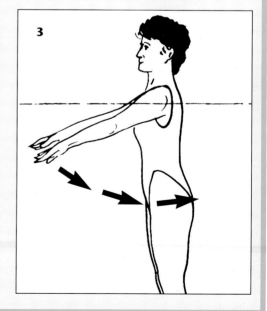

Hydrotherapy exercises

4 Using a collar and rubber ring for support, push one leg down into the water, keeping the knee straight. Repeat with the other leg.
5 Now push both legs down, again keeping the knees straight. Repeat 5 times.

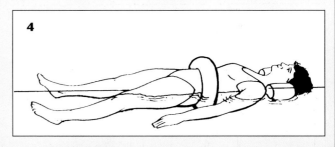

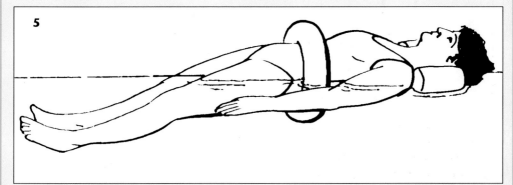

posture, which can help them to walk and sit taller and ease the pain.

Regular exercise in warm water in a hydrotherapy pool under the supervision of a physiotherapist can help relax tight muscles and joints, soothe pain and improve mobility. The buoyancy of the water helps and a gentle workout once or twice a week can have enormous benefits both physically and in mental outlook.

Your posture is important

Improving your posture may help you to straighten up, especially if you are an osteoporosis sufferer and your spine is more curved than it used to be. It helps if you are aware of your body and how you are moving: always try to 'walk tall', and swing your arms and pull your shoulders back. By correcting your posture, not only will you be able to stand up straighter but you will also look taller. You can ask your doctor to measure you twice or three times a year when you visit the surgery. Here is a quick

Exercise

checklist for correcting your posture:

1 Stand up straight. This is not as easy as it sounds, so try standing against a wall with your back resting flat on it.

2 Now pull your chin in and hopefully feel the wall against the back of your head.

3 Pull your shoulders back, your stomach in, and push your hips back. Your weight should be distributed equally on both legs.

4 You should now look more upright with a straighter spine.

Are you sitting comfortably?

Your posture is also important when you are seated. Don't slump in your chair. Sit up straight in a comfortable chair with some support for your lower back – there is less strain on the spine.

Posture

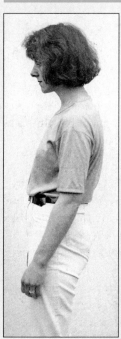
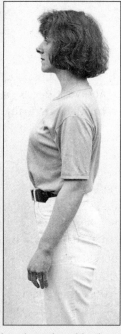

Here you can see examples of good and bad posture. Don't slump your shoulders and stick your stomach out (left). This puts strain on your back. Stand up straight (right) with shoulders back and stomach pulled in.

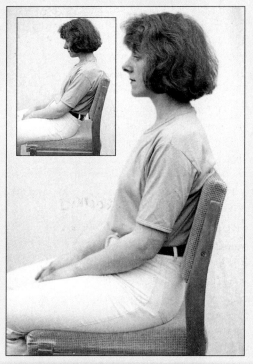

When you sit down, make sure that you sit up straight with your back well supported.

When choosing a chair, make sure that your feet are resting on the ground. They need to be supported in this way or you will increase the pressure on your spine. Your hips and bottom should be positioned well back in the chair.

Getting a good night's sleep

It is also important that your bed is comfortable and that the mattress is firm and supports your weight without sagging. This does not necessarily mean that you have to buy a really hard mattress, especially if you are used to a soft one, nor is it necessary to place a board under the mattress. Some people with osteoporosis find that sleeping on a 'bean bag'-type mattress is particularly effective in giving support and comfort.

Home exercise programme

Here is a simple programme of exercises that you can perform at home. Obviously the sort of exercises you attempt and the number of repetitions you do will depend on how fit you are, the severity of your osteoporosis and any pain you may experience. Before you start, especially if you are not very mobile and are unused to exercise, it is advisable to consult your doctor.

Safety guidelines

● Consult your doctor first before exercising.
● Start slowly – don't try too much too quickly.
● If you experience pain, stop. Don't try to work through it.
● Listen to your body and what it tells you.
● Little and often is better than a strenuous work-out once a week.
● Keep your movements smooth and fluid, moving slowly – not jerky.

General exercise rules

Start off slowly, repeating each exercise 5-10 times, depending on how you feel and your degree of suppleness. You can build up gradually to more repetitions as you get fitter and stronger.

These exercises can be performed any time and if you practise them regularly and make them part of your daily routine, they will help to improve your posture, strengthen the muscles that support the bones, and improve the mobility in your spine and joints. They may even help to reduce the rate of bone lossif performed regularly over a period of time.

Exercises lying down

If you have difficulties getting down on the floor, then you should omit the exercises shown on the following pages which are done lying down; or try doing them on a firm bed.

Exercise

Full body stretch

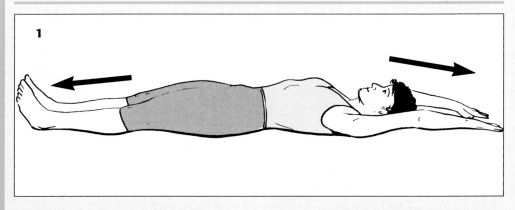

1 Stretch out as far as you can go in both directions. Try to imagine that you are making yourself longer, stretching your arms back in one direction and your feet forwards in the other direction.

2 Lower your arms to the floor by your sides, and bend your left hip and knee towards you, sliding your left foot along the floor or bed. Lower slowly and repeat with the other leg.

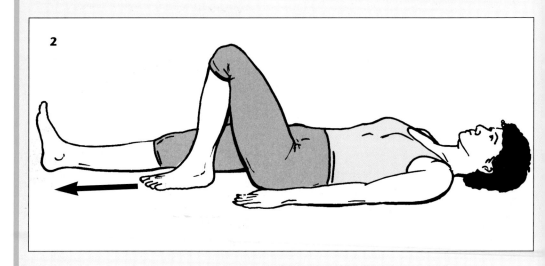

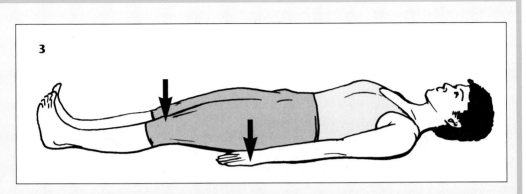

3 Keeping your back straight, push your hands and knees down, and tighten your thigh, buttock and back muscles.

4 Lying flat with your legs straight out, try to 'hitch' one leg up towards you making it shorter, and then push down to make the leg longer (inset). Repeat with the other leg.

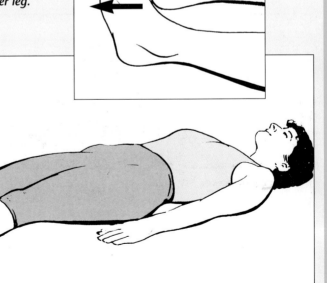

Exercise

Stretching and strengthening exercise

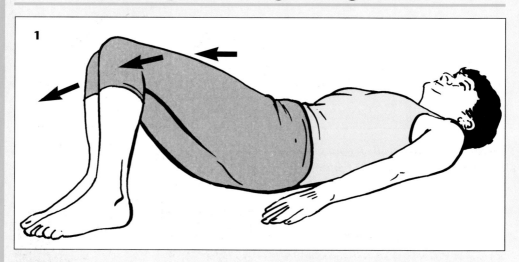

1 With your knees together, roll them first to one side and then to the other side, twisting from the waist downwards. Only twist as far as feels comfortable.

2 Put both hands in the small of your back and flatten the spine on to your hands. Hold the position briefly and then gently arch your spine away from your hands.

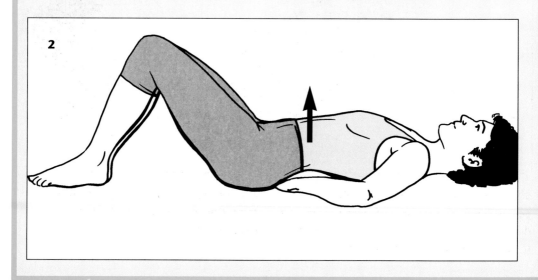

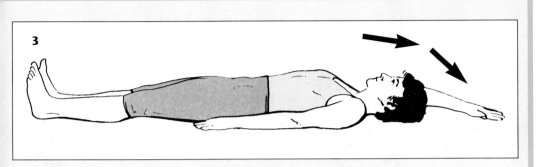

3 Stretch one arm overhead and press it on to the floor or bed. Repeat with the other arm.

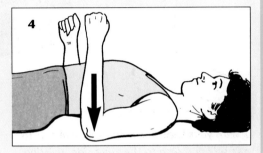

4 With your hips and shoulders flat on the floor or bed, tuck your elbows in and press them on to the floor or bed. Hold and then relax.

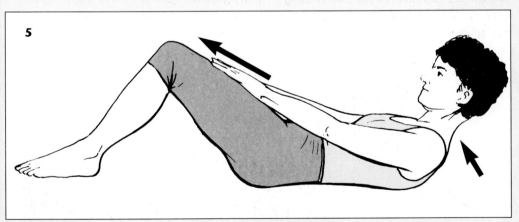

5 If you can manage it, finish off with some gentle sit-ups to strengthen the stomach muscles. Place your hands on your thighs and slide them towards the knees as you slowly lift your head and shoulders up and then gently lower them. Only do this exercise if it feels comfortable.

Exercise

Exercises on your front

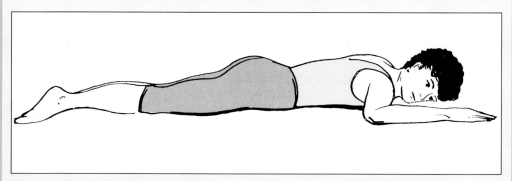

Note: You should only attempt these exercises if you can lie on your stomach comfortably with your hands positioned by your sides or resting your forehead on the palms of your hands. This may prove impossible if your spine is quite curved.

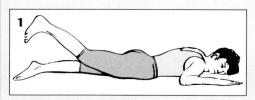

1 Lift one leg off the floor, keeping the knee straight. Lower slowly and then repeat the exercise with the other leg.

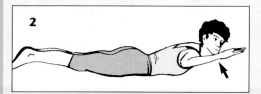

2 Lift your head and shoulders about 10cm/4 inches off the floor, and then lower them slowly. If this is painful, don't attempt this

exercise until you are more mobile. Start by lifting just your head off the floor.

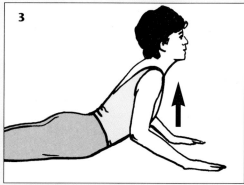

3 Place your hands on the floor with your elbows, slightly bent, by your sides as if you are going to do a press-up. Now push your hands into the floor, lifting your head and shoulders up and keeping your hips down.

Kneeling exercises

Note: *You should only attempt these exercises if you feel comfortable and well balanced on all-fours and can kneel safely.*

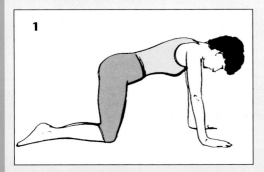

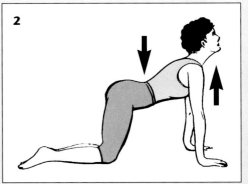

1 & 2 On all-fours, arch your back and look upwards. Return to the starting position.

3 Lift one leg off the floor and stretch it out behind you, keeping your spine straight. Lower and repeat with the other leg.

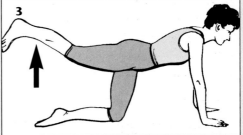

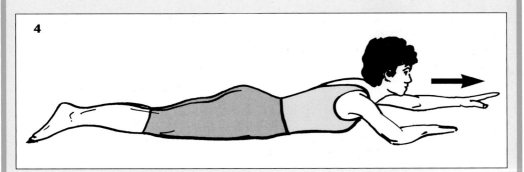

4 On all-fours, stretch one arm out in front of you and look up at your arm. Repeat with the other arm. Alternatively, you can do this exercise lying on your front.

Exercise

Seated exercises

Do these exercises seated on a chair with support in the lower back. This will help to keep you upright as you do the exercises.

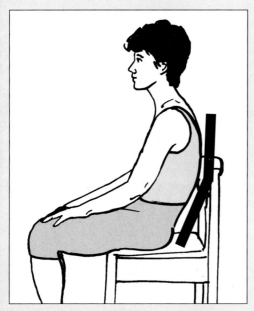

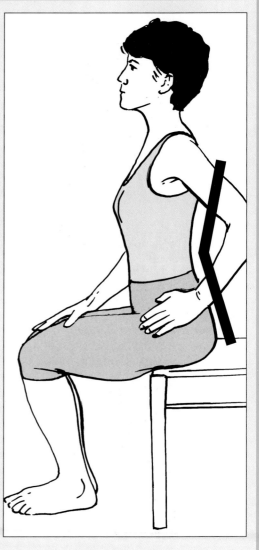

Allow the lower part of your spine to 'sag' and then straighten up to make a small curve at the base of your spine.

Seated exercises

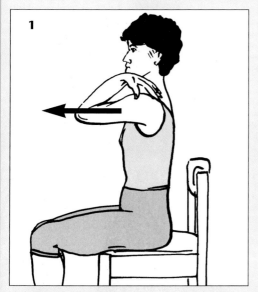

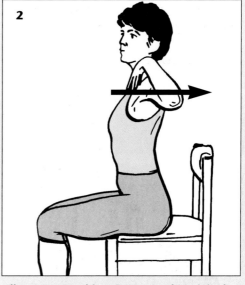

1 & 2 Rest your fingertips on your shoulders, then bring your arms forwards until your elbows are touching. Return to the original starting position. Repeat, stretching your arms out and back as you go.

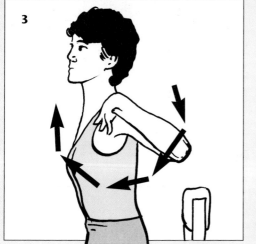

3 Still with your fingertips on your shoulders, circle your arms in large circular movements, without pushing your chin forwards.

Exercise

Standing exercises

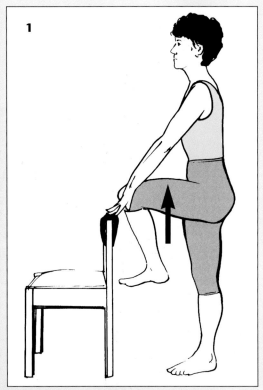

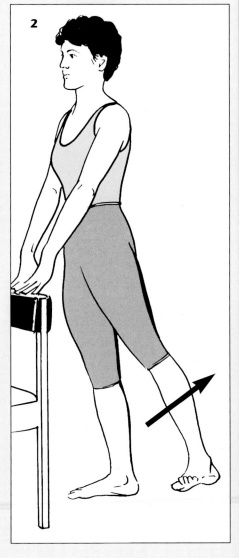

These exercises should be done holding on to a chair or, better still, a firm fixed surface such as a towel rail or washbasin.

1 Bend your right leg upwards towards your chest. Lower and repeat with the other leg.

2 Raise one leg out to the side. Return to the starting position and then repeat with the other leg.

Standing exercises

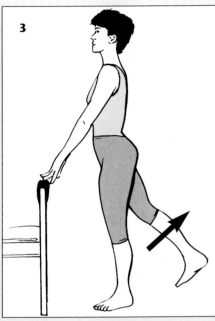

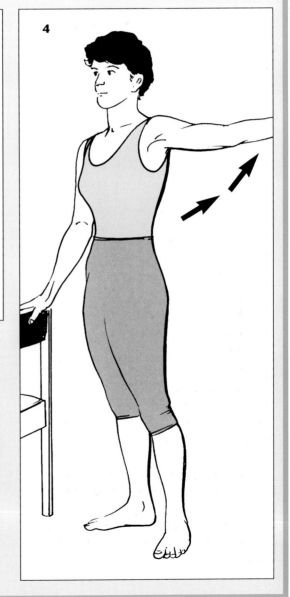

3 Raise your leg and swing it out backwards behind you, keeping the knee straight. Repeat with the other leg.

4 Stand to one side of the chair or towel rail, holding on to it with one hand. Circle your other arm steadily, and then repeat with the other hand. Keep straight and don't let your chin push forwards.

Exercise

Standing exercises

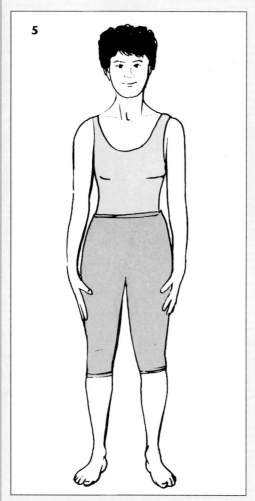

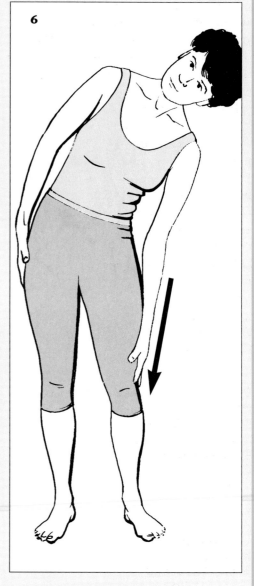

5 & 6 Standing with feet apart and your back to the wall, rest your arms by your sides. Now slide your right arm down the right leg as far as it will go. Slide back up to the middle and repeat with the left arm.

Useful addresses

National Osteoporosis Society
This is an independent and unbiased organisation with its own specialist medical advisors. It is the only registered UK charity raising funds exclusively to improve diagnosis, treatment and prevention of osteoporosis.

Hundreds of thousands have benefited from NOS advice on how to avoid osteoporosis, and many sufferers have been helped to obtain treatment. Desperately needed research, such as into osteoporosis in children, is being funded by the NOS.

The NOS has a wide range of useful literature and runs a helpline. Why not join? Write to:
National Osteoporosis Society
PO Box 10
Radstock
Bath BA3 3YB
Tel: 0761 432472
Helpline: 0761 431594

The National Dairy Council has a range of booklets which provide information on calcium in dairy products.
National Dairy Council
5-7 John Princes Street
London W1M 0AP
Tel: 071 499 7822

The Vegetarian Society
Parkdale
Dunham Road
Altrincham
Cheshire WA14 4QG
Tel: 061 928 0793

The Vegan Society
7 Battle Road
St Leonards on Sea
East Sussex TN37 7AA
Tel: 0424 427393

Overseas organisations

Australia
The Osteoporosis Foundation of Australia Incorporated
100 Miller Street
27th Floor
North Sydney 2060
Australia

Canada
Osteoporosis Society of Canada
Suite 502
76 St Claire Avenue West
Toronto M4V 1N2
Canada

Europe
European Foundation for Osteoporosis and Bone Disease
Pavillon F
Hopital Edouard Herriot
69437 Lyon Cedex 03
France

United States
National Osteoporosis Foundation
1625 Eye Street, N.W.
Suite 822
Washington D.C.
20006
USA

Index

W A R

FAMILY

OSTEOPOROSIS

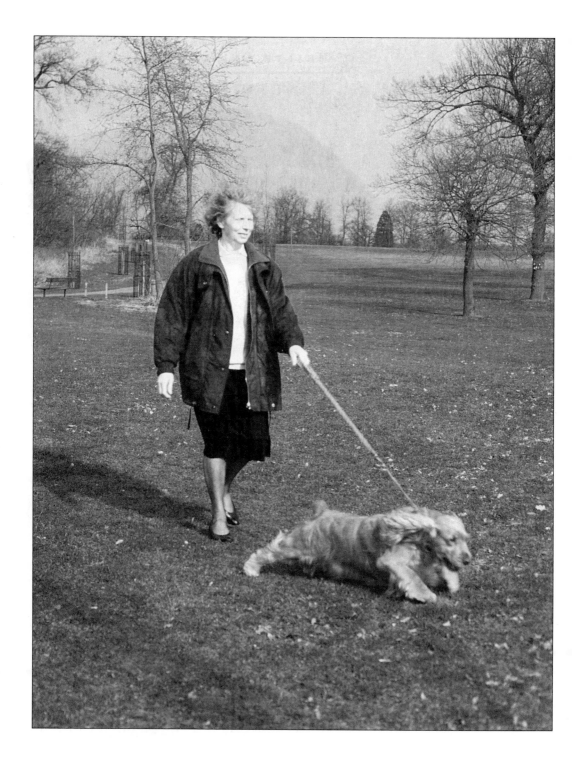